DASH DIET COOKBOOK FOR BEGINNERS

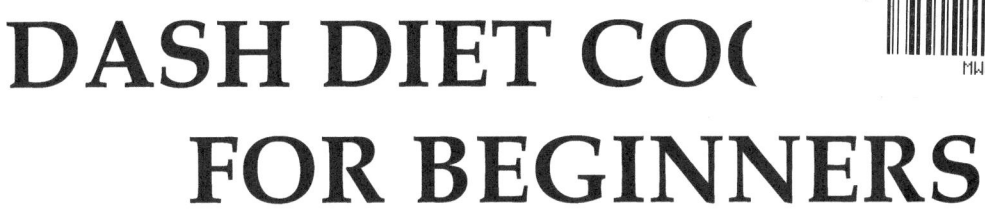

Delicious and Easy-to-Prepare Recipes Low in Sodium and High in Potassium to Manage Hypertension & Stress! A Time-Saving & Life-Simplifying 12-Week Meal Plan!

Isolde Brightwood

Copyrighted Material

© Copyright 2024 - Isolde Brightwood - All rights reserved.

No part of this publication may be reproduced, stored in a retrieval system, or transmitted in any form or by any means, electronic, mechanical, photocopying, recording, or otherwise, without prior written permission from the author or the legal copyright holder.

Legal Accountability

The publisher and the author take care in preparing this book but make no expressed or implied warranty of any kind and assume no responsibility for errors or omissions. No liability is assumed for incidental or consequential damages in connection with or arising out of the use of the information or programs contained herein.

Legal Notice

This work is protected under United States Copyright Law and is intended for the personal non-commercial use of the purchaser. Any reproduction, sharing of this material, for commercial or non-commercial purposes, without the explicit consent of the author, is strictly prohibited.

Disclaimer Notice

The material within this book is for informational purposes only and is not intended as professional advice. Efforts have been made to ensure that content is accurate and current. The author disclaims all warranties, express or implied, as to the accuracy, legality, reliability, or validity of any content within this book and will not be liable for any errors or omissions or any damages suffered from the use of this information. Readers are advised to consult with a qualified professional for advice on their specific circumstances.

By reading this book, you agree to indemnify and hold harmless the author from any claim, action, or demand arising out of or related to the use of the information herein.

Table of Contents

INTRODUCTION 7
- UNDERSTANDING HYPERTENSION: THE SILENT THREAT 7
  - *What is Hypertension* 7
  - *Why Should You Care?* 7
  - *Active steps for managing and Preventing Hypertension* 8
- THE POWER OF NUTRITION IN COMBATING HIGH BLOOD PRESSURE 9
  - *Nutrition and High Blood Pressure* 9
  - *The Role of Sodium in Hypertension: Why It Matters?* 9
- ALLOWED VS. NOT ALLOWED: A COMPREHENSIVE GUIDE 11
  - *Not Recommended Foods* 11
  - *Allowed Foods* 12
- WHY THE DASH DIET? A SCIENCE-BACKED APPROACH 13
  - *The Science Behind the DASH Diet* 13
  - *Benefits of the DASH Diet: Beyond Blood Pressure* 14
  - *Essential Ingredients for Your DASH Pantry* 15

SUNRISE SPLENDORS: BREAKFASTS TO FUEL YOUR DAY 16
- 1. SPINACH AND MUSHROOM BREAKFAST QUESADILLA 16
- 2. BANANA NUT OVERNIGHT OATS 16
- 3. BLUEBERRY PROTEIN PANCAKES 17
- 4. POACHED EGGS WITH SALSA 17
- 5. PEANUT BUTTER AND BANANA SMOOTHIE 18
- 6. VEGGIE BREAKFAST BURRITO 18
- 7. SWEET POTATO AND BLACK BEAN HASH 19
- 8. WHOLE WHEAT FRENCH TOAST WITH BERRIES 20
- 9. BREAKFAST TOFU SCRAMBLE 20
- 10. TOMATO AND BASIL OMELET 21
- 11. ALMOND BUTTER AND APPLE SANDWICH 21
- 12. QUINOA AND BERRY BREAKFAST BOWL 22
- 13. BROCCOLI AND CHEDDAR FRITTATA 22
- 14. SPINACH AND TOMATO BREAKFAST WRAP 23
- 15. CINNAMON RAISIN OATMEAL 23
- 16. WHOLE WHEAT CREPES WITH STRAWBERRIES 24
- 17. BREAKFAST MUFFIN WITH SPINACH AND FETA 25
- 18. OVERNIGHT CHIA PUDDING WITH MANGO 25
- 19. COTTAGE CHEESE AND PINEAPPLE BOWL 26
- 20. GREEK YOGURT WITH KIWI SLICES 26
- 21. SPINACH AND FETA BREAKFAST PIE 27
- 22. BREAKFAST TACOS WITH BLACK BEANS AND AVOCADO 27
- 23. OAT BRAN CEREAL WITH ALMOND MILK 28
- 24. ALMOND AND DATE BREAKFAST BARS 29
- 25. QUINOA AND SPINACH BREAKFAST CASSEROLE 29

SNIP TASTY MORSELS: HEALTHY SNACKS FOR EVERY CRAVING 31
- 26. ROASTED RED PEPPER HUMMUS WITH CARROT STICKS 31
- 27. PEAR SLICES WITH COTTAGE CHEESE 31
- 28. BAKED KALE CHIPS 32

29. Cherry Tomato and Mozzarella Skewers 32
30. Rice Cakes with Peanut Butter and Banana 33
31. Greek Yogurt with Pomegranate Seeds 33
32. Mixed Nuts (Unsalted) and Sliced Apple 33
33. Cucumber Slices with Greek Yogurt Dip 34
34. Air-Popped Popcorn 34
35. Edamame 34
36. Roasted Chickpeas 35
37. Sliced Bell Peppers with Guacamole 35
38. Watermelon Cubes 36
39. Pineapple and Cottage Cheese 36
40. Almond Butter and Banana Slices 36
41. Greek Yogurt with Papaya 37
42. Sliced Mango with Lime 37
43. Celery Sticks with Hummus and Raisins 37
44. Mixed Berries with Greek Yogurt 38
45. Apple Cinnamon Rice Cakes 38

BOWLS OF BOUNTY: HEARTWARMING SOUPS & CRISP SALADS 39

46. Quinoa and Black Bean Salad 39
47. Roasted Beet and Goat Cheese Salad 40
48. Spinach and Chickpea Salad with Lemon Vinaigrette 40
49. Mushroom Barley Soup 41
50. Greek Quinoa Salad 42
51. Roasted Butternut Squash Salad 42
52. Chicken and Vegetable Stir-Fry Soup 43
53. Spinach and Pomegranate Salad 44
54. Lentil and Vegetable Soup 44
55. Caprese Salad with Balsamic Glaze 45
56. Avocado and Quinoa Salad 45
57. Kale and Cranberry Salad 46
58. Tomato Cucumber Salad with Dill 47
59. Gazpacho with Cucumber Salsa 47
60. Roasted Garlic and White Bean Soup 48

PRIME PLATES: MEATY MAINS WITH A HEALTHY TWIST 49

61. Grilled Lemon Herb Chicken 49
62. Turkey and Spinach Stuffed Mushrooms 49
63. Beef and Broccoli Stir-Fry 50
64. Pork Tenderloin with Mustard Sauce 51
65. Chicken and Veggie Skewers with Tzatziki 51
66. Baked Turkey Meatloaf 52
67. Beef and Vegetable Stir-Fry 53
68. Lemon Garlic Chicken Thighs 54
69. Pork Chops with Apple and Cabbage 54
70. Teriyaki Chicken 55
71. Lemon Dill Turkey Breast 56
72. Beef and Pepper Stir-Fry 56
73. Herb-Crusted Pork Tenderloin 57
74. Turkey and Zucchini Meatballs 58
75. Lean Beef and Vegetable Stir-Fry 59

76. Balsamic Glazed Chicken Breast 59
77. Pork Stir-Fry with Broccoli and Snap Peas 60
78. Chicken and Mushroom Skillet 61
79. Teriyaki Turkey Burgers 62
80. Beef and Asparagus Stir-Fry 62

OCEAN'S OFFERINGS: FRESH FISH FEASTS FOR THE SOUL 64

81. Grilled Halibut with Mango Salsa 64
82. Tuna Salad Lettuce Wraps 64
83. Baked Mahi-Mahi with Lemon Butter 65
84. Shrimp and Spinach Salad 65
85. Baked Cod with Herbed Breadcrumbs 66
86. Salmon and Asparagus Foil Packets 67
87. Tuna and White Bean Salad with Lemon Dressing 67
88. Lemon Garlic Tilapia 68
89. Seared Scallops with Spinach and Tomato 68
90. Baked Snapper with Citrus Glaze 69
91. Canned Mackerel Salad 70
92. Grilled Sardines with Herbs 70
93. Tuna and Cucumber Roll-Ups 71
94. Lemon Dill Mackerel 72
95. Swordfish and Vegetable Kebabs 72
96. Baked Trout with Almond Crust 73
97. Seared Tuna with Sesame Seeds 73
98. Lemon Buttered Catfish 74
99. Sardine and Olive Tapenade 75
100. Baked Haddock with Lemon Pepper 75

PERFECT PAIRINGS: SIDES & SAUCES TO ELEVATE EVERY DISH 77

101. Roasted Cauliflower with Turmeric 77
102. Green Beans with Toasted Almonds and Lemon Zest 77
103. Sautéed Swiss Chard with Garlic 78
104. Brown Rice and Black Beans 78
105. Roasted Eggplant with Tahini Sauce 79
106. Mashed Butternut Squash 80
107. Sautéed Spinach with Pine Nuts 80
108. Steamed Artichokes with Lemon Butter 81
109. Cilantro Lime Brown Rice 81
110. Roasted Brussels Sprouts with Balsamic Glaze 82

SWEET TEMPTATIONS: GUILTLESS TREATS FOR DESSERT LOVERS 83

111. Baked Pear with Cinnamon and Almonds 83
112. Banana and Walnut Muffins 83
113. Chocolate Avocado Mousse 84
114. Apple Cinnamon Baked Oatmeal 84
115. Berry and Yogurt Parfait 85
116. Baked Peaches with Almond Crumble 86
117. Strawberry and Banana Popsicles 86
118. Lemon Poppy Seed Muffins 87
119. Chocolate Covered Almonds 87
120. Greek Yogurt and Berry Bark 88

- 121. Coconut and Chia Seed Pudding ... 88
- 122. Baked Apple Chips ... 89
- 123. Pineapple and Coconut Frozen Yogurt ... 89
- 124. Mixed Fruit Sorbet ... 90
- 125. Pumpkin and Walnut Bites ... 90

SIPS OF SERENITY: REFRESHING BEVERAGES FOR EVERY MOOD ... 92

- 126. Herbal Infusion with Mint and Ginger ... 92
- 127. Cranberry and Orange Smoothie ... 92
- 128. Cucumber and Mint Cooler ... 93
- 129. Cherry and Pomegranate Iced Tea ... 93
- 130. Kiwi and Spinach Smoothie ... 94

12-WEEK MEAL PLAN WITH DOWNLOADABLE SHOPPING LISTS ... 95

- Week 1 ... 96
- Week 2 ... 97
- Week 3 ... 98
- Week 4 ... 99
- Week 5 ... 100
- Week 6 ... 101
- Week 7 ... 102
- Week 8 ... 103
- Week 9 ... 104
- Week 10 ... 105
- Week 11 ... 106
- Week 12 ... 107

CONVERSION TABLE ... 108

INDEX ... 110

BONUSES ... 112

CONCLUSIONS AND RECOMMENDATIONS ... 113

- The Importance of the Meal Plan ... 113
- The Importance of Combining the Diet with Physical Exercises ... 114
- The Importance of Not Getting Discouraged and Always Maintaining a Positive Mindset ... 115

Introduction

Understanding Hypertension: The Silent Threat

Hypertension, commonly known as high blood pressure, is a medical condition that affects millions of people worldwide. Despite being a widespread health issue, hypertension is often referred to as the "silent threat" because it typically doesn't present noticeable symptoms until it reaches advanced stages. In this section, we will delve into what hypertension is, why you should care about it, and how you can manage and prevent this potentially life-threatening condition.

What is Hypertension

Hypertension, or high blood pressure, occurs when the force of your blood against the artery walls is consistently too high. Blood pressure represents the force exerted by blood on the arterial walls during the heart's pumping action, circulating throughout the body. Measurement is commonly in millimeters of mercury (mm Hg), presented as two values: systolic pressure (the upper number)-and diastolic pressure (the lower number):

- **Systolic pressure:** This is the pressure when your heart beats and pumps blood into your arteries
- **Diastolic pressure:** This is the pressure when your heart is at rest between beats.

A standard blood pressure reading typically falls around 120/80 mm Hg. Hypertension is identified when blood pressure consistently surpasses 130/80 mm Hg. Hypertension can be categorized into different stages based on blood pressure readings:

- **Normal**: Blood pressure is within the healthy range.
- **Elevated**: Blood pressure is higher than normal but not yet classified as hypertension.
- **Stage 1 Hypertension**: Is characterized by systolic pressure ranging from 130-139 mm Hg or diastolic pressure ranging from 80-89 mm Hg.
- **Stage 2 Hypertension**: Is identified when systolic pressure is 140 mm Hg or higher, or diastolic pressure is 90 mm Hg or higher.

Why Should You Care?

Hypertension is commonly referred to as the "silent killer" due to its ability to inflict damage on organs and elevate the risk of severe health complications without manifesting noticeable symptoms. Here are several reasons why you should care about hypertension:

1. **Increased Risk of Cardiovascular Diseases**: high blood pressure stands as a primary risk factor for heart diseases, strokes, and various cardiovascular conditions. Over time, it can cause damage on the arteries, heightening the likelihood of atherosclerosis—a process involving the narrowing and hardening of arteries—potentially culminating in heart attacks and strokes.
2. **Kidney Damage**: hypertension has the potential to harm blood vessels within the kidneys, diminishing their capacity to effectively filter waste from the blood. This deterioration can ultimately result in kidney disease or kidney failure.

3. **Brain Health**: uncontrolled hypertension can lead to cognitive decline and an increased risk of dementia. It also plays a role in the development of small vessel disease in the brain, potentially leading to strokes and cognitive impairment.
4. **Eye Problems**: elevated blood pressure can adversely affect the blood vessels in the eyes, contributing to vision issues and, in severe cases, potential blindness.
5. **Pregnancy Complications**: in pregnancy, hypertension can lead to preeclampsia, posing serious risks for both mother and baby, including premature birth and low birth weight.
6. **Quality of Life**: hypertension can result in a diminished quality of life marked by symptoms such as chest pain, fatigue, shortness of breath, and other factors that can impede daily activities.
7. **Risk of Other Diseases**: hypertension is frequently linked to additional health conditions like diabetes, obesity, and high cholesterol, thereby amplifying the overall risk of complications.

Active steps for managing and Preventing Hypertension

The good news is that hypertension is manageable and preventable. By adopting certain lifestyle changes, you can significantly reduce your risk. Here are some strategies to help you keep your blood pressure in check:

1. **Healthy Diet**: adopt a diet rich in whole grains, lean proteins, fruits, vegetables, and low-fat dairy products. Cut down on sodium intake and restrict processed foods, known for their high salt content.
2. **Regular Exercise**: engage in regular physical activity. Aim for at least 150 minutes of moderate-intensity exercise or 75 minutes of vigorous-intensity exercise per week. Exercise helps lower blood pressure and improve overall cardiovascular health.
3. **Maintain a Healthy Weight**: If you're overweight, losing even a small amount of weight can make a significant difference in managing hypertension.
4. **Limit Alcohol**: excessive alcohol consumption can raise blood pressure. Limit your alcohol intake or, ideally, avoid it altogether.
5. **Quit Smoking**: smoking has the potential to narrow blood vessels and increase blood pressure. Quitting smoking is a pivotal measure in lowering the risk of hypertension.
6. **Stress Management**: employ stress-reduction practices such as meditation, deep breathing, yoga, or mindfulness to alleviate stress levels, a factor contributing to hypertension.
7. **Medication**: If lifestyle changes alone aren't enough, your healthcare provider may prescribe medication to lower your blood pressure. It's essential to take these medications as prescribed and follow up with your doctor regularly.
8. **Regular Check-ups**: schedule regular visits to your healthcare provider, even if you feel well. Consistent monitoring of blood pressure and overall health is essential for the early detection and effective management of hypertension.

The Power of Nutrition in Combating High Blood Pressure

Although genetics and lifestyle choices contribute significantly to its onset, the role of nutrition is pivotal in addressing and managing hypertension effectively. Here, we will delve into the positive impact of nutrition in managing and preventing high blood pressure, with a particular focus on the role of sodium and why it matters.

Nutrition and High Blood Pressure

Nutrition plays a pivotal role in managing high blood pressure. The foods we consume can either contribute to elevated blood pressure or help keep it in check. Here are several crucial ways in which nutrition can have a positive impact on elevated blood pressure:

1. **Balanced Diet**: a balanced diet rich in whole grains, lean proteins, fruits, vegetables, and low-fat dairy products provides essential nutrients and helps maintain a healthy weight. These foods are naturally low in sodium and high in potassium, both of which play crucial roles in blood pressure regulation.
2. **Sodium Reduction**: excessive sodium intake is a significant contributor to high blood pressure. Reducing sodium in the diet can lead to lower blood pressure levels, especially in individuals who are salt-sensitive.
3. **Potassium Intake**: potassium helps counter the effects of sodium by relaxing blood vessel walls and excreting excess sodium through urine. Incorporating potassium-rich foods into your diet can contribute to the reduction of blood pressure.
4. **Healthy Fats**: replacing saturated and trans fats with healthier fats like monounsaturated and polyunsaturated fats can have a positive impact on blood pressure and overall cardiovascular health.
5. **Weight Management**: Sustaining a healthy weight by practicing proper nutrition and portion control can play a substantial role in reducing blood pressure.

The Role of Sodium in Hypertension: Why It Matters?

Sodium is a mineral that is essential for various bodily functions, including maintaining proper fluid balance, transmitting nerve signals, and supporting muscle contractions. However, too much sodium in the diet can have detrimental effects on blood pressure, as it causes the body to retain excess water, increasing the volume of blood in the arteries and ultimately raising blood pressure. Here are several reasons why sodium matters in the context of high blood pressure:

1. **Blood Pressure Regulation**: sodium plays a central role in regulating blood pressure. When there's a high concentration of sodium in the blood, the body holds onto more water to dilute the sodium levels. This, in turn, increases the volume of blood in the arteries, leading to higher blood pressure.
2. **Salt Sensitivity**: not everyone responds to sodium intake in the same way. Certain people have a higher sensitivity to salt, which means their blood pressure rises more significantly in response to increased sodium intake. Salt sensitivity is more common in people with hypertension, African Americans, and older adults.
3. **Increased Risk of Hypertension**: excessive sodium intake is a well-established risk factor for the development of hypertension. Reducing sodium consumption can help prevent hypertension and lower blood pressure in individuals with the condition.

4. **Atherosclerosis**: high sodium intake is associated with the development of atherosclerosis, a condition characterized by the narrowing and hardening of arteries. Atherosclerosis has the potential to result in heart attacks, strokes, and various other cardiovascular complications.
5. **Kidney Function**: the kidneys play a vital role in maintaining the balance of sodium in the body. Over time, high sodium intake can damage the kidneys, impairing their ability to filter waste from the blood and regulate blood pressure.

Effective Strategies to Reduce Sodium Intake for Blood Pressure Control

Reducing sodium intake is a key strategy in managing and preventing high blood pressure. Here are some practical tips to help you lower your sodium consumption:

1. **Read Food Labels**: scrutinize the nutrition labels on packaged foods to assess their sodium content. Stay alert to concealed sources of sodium, such as monosodium glutamate (MSG), sodium bicarbonate (baking soda), and sodium nitrate or nitrite.
2. **Cook at Home**: preparing meals at home provides you with the ability to regulate the amount of salt added to your dishes. Use herbs, spices, and various flavor enhancers to improve your food's taste without relying on too much salt.
3. **Choose Low-Sodium Products**: opt for low-sodium or sodium-free versions of condiments, canned vegetables, soups, and other processed foods when available.
4. **Limit Processed Foods**: processed and prepackaged foods tend to be high in sodium. Reduce your consumption of items like frozen meals, instant noodles, and canned goods.
5. **Be Cautious When Eating Out**: when dining at restaurants, request that your food be prepared with less salt or ask for sauces and dressings on the side so you can control how much you use.
6. **Rinse Canned Foods**: If you use canned vegetables or beans, rinse them thoroughly under running water to remove some of the salt. Rinsing canned foods, such as vegetables or beans, under running water can reduce the sodium content by up to 40%. This simple step helps to significantly decrease salt intake without compromising the flavor of the food.
7. **Choose Fresh Foods**: incorporate lean meats, fresh fruits & vegetables, and whole grains into your diet. These foods are naturally low in sodium.
8. **Limit Fast Food**: fast-food items are often loaded with sodium. Reducing your consumption of fast food can have a significant impact on sodium intake.
9. **Use Alternative Seasonings**: experiment with alternative seasonings like garlic, lemon juice, vinegar, and various herbs and spices to flavor your dishes.
10. **Stay Hydrated**: drinking plenty of water can help flush excess sodium from your body.

Allowed vs. Not Allowed: A Comprehensive Guide

Making the right food choices is crucial for maintaining good health and well-being. Here, we will explore common foods that are considered "allowed" and "not allowed" for a balanced and health-conscious diet. It's important to note that this categorization is not about creating strict rules but rather helping you make informed choices that can positively impact your health and quality of life.

In the table below, we provide a list of common, healthy, and allowed foods that can replace equivalent unhealthy and forbidden foods. This can serve as a handy reference for making healthier dietary choices.

Not Recommended Foods	Allowed Foods
Sugary Beverages	Water, herbal tea
Soda and carbonated drinks	Sparkling water, seltzer
Candy and sweets	Fresh fruit, dried fruit
Processed snacks (chips, crackers, etc.)	Nuts, seeds, rice cakes, vegetable sticks
Deep-fried foods (French fries, fried chicken, etc.)	Baked or grilled lean protein (chicken, fish)
Fast food burgers and fries	Homemade burgers with lean beef or turkey
Highly processed and sugary cereals	Whole grains (brown rice, oatmeal, whole wheat
Processed deli meats and sausages	Freshly cooked lean meats, poultry, or tofu
Sugary breakfast pastries	Oatmeal, whole-grain muffins
White bread and bagels	Whole-grain bread, whole-grain bagels
Full-fat dairy products	Low-fat or non-fat dairy products
Sugary yogurt and desserts	Plain Greek yogurt, yogurt with fresh fruit
Sugary condiments (ketchup, barbecue sauce)	Herbs, spices, vinegar-based sauces
Highly processed frozen dinners	Frozen vegetables, whole-food frozen meals
Sugar-laden sauces (e.g., sweet and sour sauce)	Homemade sauces with minimal added sugar
Sugary energy drinks and sports drinks	Green tea, herbal tea, homemade smoothies
High-sugar salad dressings	Homemade vinaigrettes, olive oil-based dressings
Sugary canned fruit and fruit juices	Fresh, frozen, or canned fruit in natural juice

Now, let's delve deeper into why these substitutions are recommended and why certain foods are classified as "not allowed" in a balanced diet.

Not Recommended Foods
1. **Sugary Beverages**: sugary drinks like soda, fruit juices, and energy drinks are high in added sugars and provide little to no nutritional value. They can lead to weight gain, increase the risk of type 2 diabetes, and have a negative impact on dental health.
2. **Candy and Sweets**: these are typically high in refined sugars, providing empty calories and contributing to weight gain, insulin resistance, and dental problems.

3. **Processed Snacks**: chips, crackers, and other processed snacks are often loaded with unhealthy trans fats, excessive sodium, and empty calories. They can lead to weight gain and cardiovascular issues.
4. **Deep-Fried Foods and Fast Food Options:** Deep-fried items, including French fries and fried chicken, along with fast food burgers and fries, are loaded with unhealthy trans fats, saturated fats, sodium, and excess calories. Their regular consumption contributes to obesity, heart disease, and increases the risk of chronic diseases due to high levels of unhealthy fats and added sugars.
5. **Highly Processed and Sugary Cereals**: many breakfast cereals are laden with added sugars and lack essential nutrients, potentially causing fluctuations in blood sugar levels.
6. **Processed Deli Meats and Sausages**: these processed meats often contain unhealthy additives, preservatives, and high levels of sodium and saturated fats. Regular consumption is associated with an increased risk of heart disease and certain cancers.
7. **Sugary Breakfast Pastries**: pastries like doughnuts and sweet rolls are high in added sugars and unhealthy fats. They provide little satiety and can lead to weight gain.
8. **White Bread and Bagels**: made from refined grains, white bread and bagels lack the fiber and nutrients present in whole grains, potentially causing rapid spikes in blood sugar levels.
9. **Full-Fat Dairy Products**: while dairy can be part of a healthy diet, full-fat dairy products can be high in saturated fats, which may contribute to heart disease when consumed in excess.
10. **Sugary Yogurt and Desserts**: flavored yogurts and dessert items often contain substantial added sugars, contributing to weight gain and blood sugar issues.
11. **Sugary Condiments**: condiments like ketchup and sweet barbecue sauce can add unnecessary sugar and calories to meals.
12. **Highly Processed Frozen Dinners**: frozen dinners are often high in sodium, preservatives, and unhealthy fats. They are typically lacking in essential nutrients.
13. **Sugar-Laden Sauces**: sauces like sweet and sour sauce can be loaded with added sugars, potentially contributing to excessive calorie intake.
14. **Sugary Canned Fruit:** canned fruit in syrup often have added sugars and lack the fiber found in whole fruits.

Allowed Foods
1. **Water, Sparkling Water, and Seltzer:** Maintain hydration with water and fizzy alternatives like sparkling water or seltzer, avoiding added sugars or empty calories.
2. **Fresh, Frozen, Dried Fruit, and Canned Fruit in Natural Juice:** Opt for a variety of fruits rich in vitamins, minerals, and fiber. Choose fruits without added sugars, and consider dried fruits in moderation for a convenient snack.
3. **Nuts, Seeds, Rice Cakes, and Vegetable Sticks:** These provide healthy fats, fiber, and protein, perfect for satisfying hunger between meals.
4. **Baked or Grilled Lean Protein and Homemade Burgers:** Include lean meats, poultry, tofu, and homemade burgers using lean beef or turkey. This approach minimizes excessive fats and allows for healthier cooking methods.

5. **Whole Grains, Whole-Grain Products, and Oatmeal:** Embrace brown rice, oatmeal, whole wheat bread, and whole-grain muffins for their fiber and nutrients, ensuring satiety and steady energy levels.
6. **Low-Fat or Non-Fat Dairy Products and Greek Yogurt:** Choose dairy options with reduced fat and pair plain Greek yogurt with fresh fruit for a protein-rich, naturally sweetened treat.
7. **Herbs, Spices, Vinegar-Based Sauces, and Homemade Dressings:** Enhance meals with natural seasonings and create your own dressings with olive oil to avoid added sugars and unhealthy fats.
8. **Frozen Vegetables and Whole-Food Frozen Meals**: Opt for frozen vegetables and whole-food based frozen meals for convenience without sacrificing nutritional value.
9. **Green Tea, Herbal Tea, and Homemade Smoothies:** Enjoy these beverages for their flavors and hydration benefits, steering clear of the excessive sugars found in commercial energy drinks and sports drinks.

Making informed choices about the foods we consume can exert a substantial influence on our health. While the "not allowed" foods in this guide are not necessarily off-limits, they should be consumed in moderation to promote overall well-being. By incorporating more "allowed" foods into your diet, you can enjoy a balanced and nutritious way of eating that supports your health goals. Remember that small, sustainable changes in your food choices can lead to long-term improvements in your health and quality of life.

Why the DASH Diet? A Science-Backed Approach

The DASH diet, short for Dietary Approaches to Stop Hypertension, is a scientifically supported nutritional approach acknowledged for its efficacy in controlling and preventing high blood pressure. Formulated by the National Heart, Lung, & Blood Institute (NHLBI), the DASH diet not only proves beneficial for blood pressure management but also provides a diverse array of health benefits. Here, we will explore why the DASH diet is a science-backed approach to nutrition, the benefits it provides beyond blood pressure management, and the essential ingredients you should stock in your DASH pantry.

The Science Behind the DASH Diet

The DASH diet was created based on extensive research that aimed to identify dietary patterns that could effectively lower blood pressure and reduce the risk of hypertension-related complications. Here are some key aspects of the science behind the DASH diet:

1. **Low in Sodium**: one of the primary factors contributing to high blood pressure is excessive sodium intake. The DASH diet is designed to be low in sodium, typically restricting daily sodium intake to 2,300 milligrams or less, with an even lower target of 1,500 milligrams for individuals who are particularly salt-sensitive or at a higher risk of hypertension.
2. **Rich in Nutrients**: the DASH diet emphasizes the consumption of nutrient-dense foods that provide essential vitamins, minerals, and dietary fiber. It encourages the intake of fruits, vegetables, whole grains, lean proteins, and low-fat dairy products, all of which are packed with beneficial nutrients.
3. **Balanced Macronutrients**: the DASH diet promotes a balanced distribution of macronutrients. It suggests a diet that is moderate in carbohydrates, moderate in protein, and low in total fat and saturated fat. This balance helps improve overall cardiovascular health.

4. **Emphasis on Potassium**: potassium is a crucial mineral that mitigates the impact of sodium on blood pressure. The DASH diet encourages the consumption of potassium-rich foods like bananas, oranges, potatoes, and spinach.
5. **Evidence-Based Results**: the DASH diet has been tested in numerous clinical trials and has consistently shown its effectiveness in reducing blood pressure. These trials have demonstrated that the diet can significantly lower both systolic and diastolic blood pressure levels. One of the landmark studies supporting the DASH diet is the original DASH trial conducted in 1997. This research demonstrated that the DASH diet significantly lowers blood pressure in individuals with and without hypertension, showcasing its effectiveness as a dietary strategy for blood pressure management.

Benefits of the DASH Diet: Beyond Blood Pressure

While the primary goal of the DASH diet is to manage and prevent high blood pressure, its positive impact extends beyond blood pressure control. Here are some extra health advantages linked to the DASH diet:
1. **Heart Health**: the DASH diet is heart-healthy due to its emphasis on low-sodium, low-saturated fat, and nutrient-dense foods. It helps reduce the risk of heart disease by improving cholesterol levels, reducing inflammation, and supporting overall cardiovascular health.
2. **Weight Management**: the DASH diet can assist with weight management or weight loss due to its focus on whole, filling foods. By promoting satiety and preventing overeating, it can help individuals achieve and maintain a healthy weight.
3. **Reduced Risk of Stroke**: in addition to lowering blood pressure, the DASH diet can decrease the risk of stroke, a common complication of hypertension. Its nutrient-rich foods support optimal brain health and reduce the likelihood of stroke events.
4. **Diabetes Prevention**: the DASH diet may help prevent or manage type 2 diabetes. Its balanced macronutrient distribution and emphasis on whole grains and vegetables can help stabilize blood sugar levels.
5. **Improved Digestive Health**: the high fiber content in the DASH diet aids in digestive health by promoting regular bowel movements and preventing constipation. It may also reduce the risk of developing gastrointestinal disorders.
6. **Cancer Prevention**: Although not the primary focus, the DASH diet's emphasis on fruits, vegetables, and whole grains may help reduce the risk of some cancers due to their rich antioxidant content, but it is important to note that more research is needed to establish a direct link between diet and cancer risk reduction.
7. **Bone Health**: low-fat dairy products, a component of the DASH diet, provide essential calcium and vitamin D, supporting strong and healthy bones.
8. **Enhanced Nutrient Intake**: the DASH diet encourages the consumption of a wide variety of nutrient-rich foods, ensuring individuals receive a broad spectrum of vitamins and minerals for optimal health.
9. **Reduced Risk of Kidney Stones**: the DASH diet's emphasis on increased fluid intake and the consumption of certain fruits and vegetables can help reduce the risk of kidney stone formation.
10. **Long-Term Health**: adopting the DASH diet as a long-term dietary pattern can lead to lasting health benefits. Its sustainability makes it a practical choice for those looking to improve their overall well-being.

Essential Ingredients for Your DASH Pantry

To fully embrace the DASH diet and its health benefits, it's essential to stock your pantry with the right ingredients. Here's a list of essential items to keep on hand:

1. **Fresh Fruits**: choose a variety of fresh fruits, such as apples, berries, oranges, and bananas, to meet your daily fruit intake goals.
2. **Fresh Vegetables**: stock up on a wide range of fresh vegetables, including leafy greens, carrots, broccoli, and bell peppers.
3. **Whole Grains**: choose whole wheat pasta, whole grains such as brown rice, quinoa, and whole grain bread as substitutes for refined grains.
4. **Lean Proteins**: stock up on sources of lean protein like skinless poultry, fish, tofu, and legumes in your pantry and freezer.
5. **Low-Fat or Non-Fat Dairy**: choose low-fat or non-fat dairy products like milk, yogurt, and cheese to meet your calcium and protein needs.
6. **Nuts and Seeds**: keep a selection of nuts (e.g., almonds, walnuts) and seeds (e.g., chia seeds, flaxseeds) for added nutrients and healthy fats.
7. **Beans and Lentils**: keep canned or dried beans and lentils in stock; they serve as excellent sources of plant-based protein and fiber.
8. **Herbs and Spices**: build a collection of herbs and spices to season your dishes without relying on excessive salt. Consider options like basil, oregano, garlic, and turmeric. If fresh herbs are not available, have dried herbs and spices like thyme, rosemary, and cumin to season your dishes.
9. **Olive Oil**: Opt for extra-virgin olive oil as your main cooking oil due to its heart-friendly monounsaturated fats.
10. **Canned Tomatoes**: keep canned tomatoes, tomato sauce, or tomato paste for use in various recipes like soups, sauces, and stews.
11. **Low-Sodium Broth**: stock low-sodium vegetable or chicken broth to enhance the flavor of your dishes without excess sodium.
12. **Oats**: include oats for making oatmeal and adding fiber to baked goods.
13. **Vinegar**: have vinegar options like balsamic, apple cider, and red wine vinegar on hand for salad dressings and marinades.
14. **Frozen Vegetables**: alongside fresh vegetables, maintain an assortment of frozen vegetables in your freezer for added convenience.
15. **Fruit and Vegetable Juices**: choose 100% fruit and vegetable juices without added sugars for added nutrients.
16. **Nut and Fruit Bars**: stock healthy snack options like nut and fruit bars for on-the-go choices that align with the DASH diet principles.

By having these essential ingredients readily available in your pantry, you'll be better equipped to prepare DASH-friendly meals and snacks that promote overall health and well-being.

Note: The foods suggested in the following recipes can be consumed in varying amounts or not consumed at all for those with hypertension. Always consult your doctor for added precaution.

Sunrise Splendors: Breakfasts to Fuel Your Day

1. Spinach and Mushroom Breakfast Quesadilla

Preparation time: 10 minutes

Cooking time: 10 minutes

Servings: 2

Ingredients:

- 4 whole-grain tortillas
- 1 cup fresh spinach, chopped
- 1 cup mushrooms, sliced
- 1 cup egg whites (or whole eggs)
- 1/2 cup low-fat shredded cheese
- Salsa (no added salt) for serving

Directions:

1. Sauté the mushrooms in a non-stick skillet until they are tender. Then, add the chopped spinach and cook until it wilts.
2. Whisk the egg whites (or whole eggs) in a separate bowl. Pour this mixture over the vegetables in the skillet and cook until the eggs are set.
3. Lay a tortilla in the skillet. Spoon half of the egg and vegetable mixture onto the tortilla, then sprinkle with cheese. Top with another tortilla.
4. Cook the quesadilla for a few minutes on each side, until the tortilla turns crispy and the cheese has melted.
5. Repeat the process for the second quesadilla. Once cooked, cut it into wedges and serve with salsa.

Per serving: Calories: 300kcal; Saturated fat: 3g; Sugar: 2g; Sodium: 250mg

2. Banana Nut Overnight Oats

Preparation time: 5 minutes

Cooking time: 0 minutes

Servings: 2

Ingredients:

- 1 cup old-fashioned oats
- 1 cup unsweetened almond milk
- 1 large banana, mashed
- 2 tablespoons chopped nuts (e.g., almonds or walnuts)
- 1/2 teaspoon cinnamon
- 1 teaspoon honey (optional)

Directions:
1. In a bowl, combine the oats, almond milk, mashed banana, chopped nuts, and cinnamon.
2. Evenly divide the mixture into two jars or containers and secure the lids.
3. Refrigerate overnight.
4. Before serving, optionally drizzle honey over the oats for added sweetness.

Per serving: Calories: 250kcal; Saturated fat: 1g; Sugar: 8g; Sodium: 80mg

3. Blueberry Protein Pancakes

Preparation time: 10 minutes
Cooking time: 10 minutes
Servings: 2
Ingredients:

- 1 cup whole wheat flour
- 1 scoop (about 20g) unflavored protein powder
- 1 tablespoon baking powder
- 1 cup unsweetened almond milk
- 1 egg
- 1 cup fresh or frozen blueberries

Directions:
1. Whisk together the whole wheat flour, protein powder, and baking powder in a bow.
2. Add the almond milk and egg to the dry ingredients, stirring until just combined.
3. Gently fold in blueberries.
4. Heat a non-stick skillet over medium heat. Spoon the batter onto the skillet to form pancakes.
5. Cook the pancakes until bubbles form on the surface. Then flip them and cook the other side until golden brown.

Per serving: Calories: 350kcal; Saturated fat: 1g; Sugar: 4g; Sodium: 200mg

4. Poached Eggs with Salsa

Preparation time: 5 minutes
Cooking time: 5 minutes
Servings: 2
Ingredients:

- 4 large eggs
- 1 cup salsa (no added salt)
- Fresh cilantro for garnish

Directions:
1. Bring a pot of water to a simmer.
2. Crack each egg into a separate small bowl.
3. Gently slide each egg into the simmering water. Poach for 3-4 minutes, or until the egg whites are set.
4. Using a slotted spoon, carefully remove the poached eggs and place them on a plate lined with paper towels to drain excess water.
5. Serve the poached eggs over the salsa and garnish with fresh cilantro.

Per serving: Calories: 200kcal; Saturated fat: 2g; Sugar: 6g; Sodium: 300mg

5. Peanut Butter and Banana Smoothie

Preparation time: 5 minutes
Cooking time: 0 minutes
Servings: 2
Ingredients:

- 2 ripe bananas
- 2 tablespoons natural peanut butter
- 1 cup plain Greek yogurt (unsweetened)
- 1 cup unsweetened almond milk
- Ice cubes (optional)

Directions:
1. Combine the bananas, peanut butter, Greek yogurt, and almond milk in a blender.
2. Blend until the mixture becomes smooth.
3. If desired, add ice cubes and blend again to achieve your preferred consistency.
4. Pour the smoothie into glasses and serve.

Per serving: Calories: 300kcal; Saturated fat: 2g; Sugar: 12g; Sodium: 120mg

6. Veggie Breakfast Burrito

Preparation time: 10 minutes
Cooking time: 10 minutes
Servings: 2
Ingredients:

- 4 whole-grain tortillas
- 4 large eggs, scrambled
- 1 cup black beans, that is drained and rinsed
- 1 cup bell peppers, diced
- 1 cup tomatoes, diced

- 1/2 cup reduced-fat shredded cheese
- Salsa (no added salt) for serving

Directions:
1. Sauté the bell peppers in a non-stick skillet until they are slightly tender.
2. Add the black beans and tomatoes to the skillet and heat through.
3. Scramble the eggs in a separate pan until they are fully cooked.
4. Warm the tortillas in a dry skillet or microwave.
5. Assemble the burritos by layering the scrambled eggs, vegetable mixture, and cheese on each tortilla. Then, roll up the tortillas to enclose the filling.
6. Serve with salsa on the side.

Per serving: Calories: 400kcal; Saturated fat: 3g; Sugar: 4g; Sodium: 350mg

7. Sweet Potato and Black Bean Hash

Preparation time: 15 minutes

Cooking time: 20 minutes

Servings: 2

Ingredients:

- 2 medium sweet potatoes, peeled and diced
- 1 can (15 oz) black beans, that is drained and rinsed
- 1 cup bell peppers, diced
- 1 cup red onion, diced
- 1 teaspoon ground cumin
- 1 teaspoon chili powder
- Olive oil spray
- Salt and pepper to taste
- Fresh cilantro for garnish

Directions:
1. Heat the olive oil spray in a large skillet over medium heat.
2. Add the sweet potatoes, black beans, bell peppers, and red onion to the skillet.
3. Season with cumin, chili powder, salt, and pepper. Cook until the sweet potatoes are tender, stirring occasionally.
4. Serve the hash topped with fresh cilantro.

Per serving: Calories: 350kcal; Saturated fat: 1g; Sugar: 8g; Sodium: 300mg

8. Whole Wheat French Toast with Berries

Preparation time: 10 minutes

Cooking time: 10 minutes

Servings: 2

Ingredients:

- 4 slices whole wheat bread
- 2 large eggs
- 1/2 cup skim milk
- 1 teaspoon vanilla extract
- 1/2 teaspoon cinnamon
- Cooking spray
- Fresh berries for topping

Directions:

1. Whisk together the eggs, milk, vanilla extract, and cinnamon in a shallow bowl.
2. Heat a non-stick skillet over medium heat and coat it with cooking spray.
3. Dip each slice of bread into the egg mixture, coating both sides, and then place it in the skillet.
4. Cook each slice until it is golden brown on each side.
5. Top the French toast with fresh berries before serving.

Per serving: Calories: 250kcal; Saturated fat: 1g; Sugar: 6g; Sodium: 200mg

9. Breakfast Tofu Scramble

Preparation time: 10 minutes

Cooking time: 10 minutes

Servings: 2

Ingredients:

- 1 block (14 oz) extra-firm tofu, crumbled
- 1 tablespoon olive oil
- 1/2 cup bell peppers, diced
- 1/2 cup cherry tomatoes, halved
- 1/4 cup red onion, finely chopped
- 2 cloves garlic, minced
- 1 teaspoon turmeric (for color)
- Salt and pepper to taste
- Fresh parsley for garnish

Directions:

1. Heat the olive oil in a skillet over medium heat.
2. Add the red onion and garlic to the skillet, and sauté until they are softened.

3. Add the crumbled tofu and turmeric to the skillet, stirring to combine.
4. Add the bell peppers and cherry tomatoes, cooking until the vegetables are tender.
5. Season with salt and pepper to taste.
6. Garnish with fresh parsley before serving.

Per serving: Calories: 250kcal; Saturated fat: 2g; Sugar: 2g; Sodium: 150mg

10. Tomato and Basil Omelet

Preparation time: 10 minutes
Cooking time: 5 minutes
Servings: 2
Ingredients:

- 4 large eggs
- 1/2 cup cherry tomatoes, halved
- 2 tablespoons fresh basil, chopped
- Salt and pepper to taste
- Cooking spray

Directions:

1. Whisk the eggs in a bowl until well combined.
2. Heat a non-stick skillet over medium heat and coat it with cooking spray.
3. Pour the eggs into the skillet, swirling the skillet to spread the eggs evenly.
4. Sprinkle the cherry tomatoes and fresh basil over one half of the omelet.
5. Cook until the edges of the omelet are set, then carefully fold it in half.
6. Season with salt and pepper to taste, then serve the omelet hot.

Per serving: Calories: 180kcal; Saturated fat: 4g; Sugar: 2g; Sodium: 150mg

11. Almond Butter and Apple Sandwich

Preparation time: 5 minutes
Cooking time: 0 minutes
Servings: 1
Ingredients:

- 2 slices whole grain bread
- 2 tablespoons almond butter (no added sugar)
- 1/2 apple, thinly sliced

Directions:

1. Spread the almond butter evenly on one side of each bread slice.
2. Arrange the apple slices evenly on top of one of the almond butter-coated bread slices.
3. Place the second slice of bread on top, with the almond butter side facing the apple slices.

4. Press gently to make a sandwich.
5. Cut the sandwich in half and serve.

Per serving: Calories: 350kcal; Saturated fat: 2g; Sugar: 12g; Sodium: 200mg

12. Quinoa and Berry Breakfast Bowl

Preparation time: 15 minutes

Cooking time: 15 minutes (for quinoa)

Servings: 2

Ingredients:

- 1 cup cooked quinoa
- 1 cup mixed berries (such as blueberries, strawberries, raspberries)
- 1/4 cup almonds, sliced
- 1 tablespoon honey
- 1/2 cup Greek yogurt (unsweetened)

Directions:

1. In a bowl, create a layer of cooked quinoa.
2. Top the quinoa with mixed berries and sliced almonds.
3. Drizzle honey over the berries and quinoa for added sweetness.
4. Add a dollop of Greek yogurt on top.
5. Gently mix the ingredients before eating to combine the flavors.

Per serving: Calories: 300kcal; Saturated fat: 1g; Sugar: 12g; Sodium: 50mg

13. Broccoli and Cheddar Frittata

Preparation time: 10 minutes

Cooking time: 20 minutes

Servings: 2

Ingredients:

- 4 large eggs
- 1 cup broccoli florets, steamed and chopped
- 1/2 cup cheddar cheese, shredded
- 1/4 cup milk
- Salt and pepper to taste
- Cooking spray

Directions:

1. Preheat the oven to 350°F.
2. Whisk together the eggs, milk, salt, and pepper in a bowl.
3. Coat an oven-safe skillet with cooking spray and heat it over medium heat.

4. Pour the egg mixture into the skillet and evenly distribute the broccoli and cheddar throughout.
5. Cook on the stove for a few minutes until the edges of the frittata start to set.
6. Transfer the skillet to the preheated oven and bake for 15 minutes, or until the frittata is fully set and golden on top.
7. Slice and serve.

Per serving: Calories: 300kcal; Saturated fat: 7g; Sugar: 2g; Sodium: 350mg

14. Spinach and Tomato Breakfast Wrap

Preparation time: 10 minutes
Cooking time: 5 minutes
Servings: 2
Ingredients:

- 4 whole-grain tortillas
- 4 large eggs, scrambled
- 1 cup fresh spinach, chopped
- 1 cup cherry tomatoes, halved
- 1/2 cup feta cheese, crumbled
- Salt and pepper to taste

Directions:

1. Scramble the eggs in a non-stick skillet until they are fully cooked.
2. Warm the tortillas in a dry skillet or in the microwave.
3. Assemble the wraps by layering the scrambled eggs, chopped spinach, cherry tomatoes, and feta cheese on each tortilla.
4. Season with salt and pepper to taste.
5. Roll up the tortillas to enclose the filling and serve.

Per serving: Calories: 350kcal; Saturated fat: 5g; Sugar: 2g; Sodium: 450mg

15. Cinnamon Raisin Oatmeal

Preparation time: 5 minutes
Cooking time: 5 minutes
Servings: 2
Ingredients:

- 1 cup old-fashioned oats
- 2 cups water
- 1/2 cup raisins
- 1/2 teaspoon cinnamon
- 1 tablespoon honey (optional)

- 1/4 cup almond milk (unsweetened)

Directions:
1. Bring water to a boil in a saucepan.
2. Add the oats, then reduce the heat to a simmer. Cook for 5 minutes, stirring occasionally.
3. Stir the raisins and cinnamon into the oatmeal.
4. Sweeten the oatmeal with honey if desired.
5. Serve the oatmeal with a splash of almond milk on top.

Per serving: Calories: 250kcal; Saturated fat: 0.5g; Sugar: 12g; Sodium: 10mg

16. Whole Wheat Crepes with Strawberries

Preparation time: 15 minutes

Cooking time: 20 minutes

Servings: 2

Ingredients:
- 1 cup whole wheat flour
- 1 1/2 cups milk (skim or almond)
- 2 large eggs
- 1 tablespoon honey
- 1 teaspoon vanilla extract
- Cooking spray
- 1 cup fresh strawberries, sliced
- Greek yogurt for topping

Directions:
1. Combine the whole wheat flour, milk, eggs, honey, and vanilla extract in a blender and blend until smooth.
2. Heat a non-stick skillet over medium heat and coat it with cooking spray.
3. Pour a small amount of batter into the skillet, swirling it to spread the batter thinly.
4. Cook until the edges of the crepe lift and it can be easily flipped, then cook the other side briefly.
5. Repeat the process with the remaining batter.
6. Fill each crepe with sliced strawberries and top each with a dollop of Greek yogurt.

Per serving: Calories: 350kcal; Saturated fat: 2g; Sugar: 10g; Sodium: 150mg

17. Breakfast Muffin with Spinach and Feta

Preparation time: 15 minutes
Cooking time: 20 minutes
Servings: 2
Ingredients:

- 4 large eggs
- 1 cup spinach, chopped
- 1/2 cup feta cheese, crumbled
- 1/4 cup milk
- Salt and pepper to taste
- Cooking spray

Directions:

1. Preheat the oven to 350°F.
2. Whisk together the eggs, milk, salt, and pepper in a bowl.
3. Stir the chopped spinach and feta cheese into the egg mixture.
4. Coat the muffin tin with cooking spray.
5. Evenly distribute the egg mixture among the muffin cups.
6. Bake for 15-20 minutes, or until the muffins are set and slightly golden on top.
7. Allow to cool slightly before serving.

Per serving: Calories: 250kcal; Saturated fat: 5g; Sugar: 2g; Sodium: 350mg

18. Overnight Chia Pudding with Mango

Preparation time: 5 minutes (plus chilling time)
Cooking time: 0 minutes
Servings: 2
Ingredients:

- 1/4 cup chia seeds
- 1 cup almond milk (unsweetened)
- 1 tablespoon honey
- 1/2 teaspoon vanilla extract
- 1 cup fresh mango, diced

Directions:

1. Mix the chia seeds, almond milk, honey, and vanilla extract in a jar.
2. Stir the mixture well, then refrigerate it for at least 2 hours, or overnight, to allow the chia seeds to absorb the liquid and thicken.
3. Before serving, top the chia pudding with diced mango.

Per serving: Calories: 220kcal; Saturated fat: 1g; Sugar: 18g; Sodium: 80mg

19. Cottage Cheese and Pineapple Bowl

Preparation time: 5 minutes

Cooking time: 0 minutes

Servings: 2

Ingredients:

- 1 cup low-fat cottage cheese
- 1 cup fresh pineapple chunks
- 2 tablespoons shredded coconut
- 1 tablespoon honey (optional)
- Mint leaves for garnish

Directions:

1. Evenly divide the cottage cheese between two bowls.
2. Top each bowl evenly with fresh pineapple chunks.
3. Sprinkle the shredded coconut over the pineapple in each bowl.
4. If desired, drizzle honey over each bowl.
5. Garnish each bowl with mint leaves before serving.

Per serving: Calories: 200kcal; Saturated fat: 2g; Sugar: 15g; Sodium: 350mg

20. Greek Yogurt with Kiwi Slices

Preparation time: 5 minutes

Cooking time: 0 minutes

Servings: 2

Ingredients:

- 1 cup Greek yogurt (unsweetened)
- 2 kiwi fruits, peeled and sliced
- 2 tablespoons sliced almonds
- 1 tablespoon honey (optional)

Directions:

1. Evenly distribute the Greek yogurt into two serving bowls.
2. Arrange the kiwi slices and sprinkle the sliced almonds over the yogurt in each bowl.
3. If desired, lightly drizzle honey over each bowl.
4. Serve immediately.

Per serving: Calories: 250kcal; Saturated fat: 2g; Sugar: 16g; Sodium: 80mg

21. Spinach and Feta Breakfast Pie

Preparation time: 15 minutes

Cooking time: 25 minutes

Servings: 4

Ingredients:

- 4 large eggs
- 1 cup fresh spinach, chopped
- 1/2 cup feta cheese, crumbled
- 1/4 cup milk
- Salt and pepper to taste
- Cooking spray
- 1 sheet refrigerated pie crust

Directions:

1. Preheat the oven to 375°F.
2. Roll out the pie crust and gently press it into a pie dish, making sure it fits snugly against the sides and bottom.
3. In a bowl, whisk together the eggs, milk, salt, and pepper until well combined.
4. Fold in the chopped spinach and crumbled feta cheese into the egg mixture.
5. Pour the egg mixture into the prepared pie crust, spreading it evenly.
6. Bake for 25 minutes, or until the filling is set and the crust has turned golden brown.
7. Let the pie cool slightly before slicing into portions.

Per serving: Calories: 300kcal; Saturated fat: 7g; Sugar: 2g; Sodium: 400mg

22. Breakfast Tacos with Black Beans and Avocado

Preparation time: 15 minutes

Cooking time: 10 minutes

Servings: 2

Ingredients:

- 4 small whole-grain tortillas
- 1 can (15 oz) black beans, that is drained and rinsed
- 1 teaspoon ground cumin
- 1 teaspoon chili powder
- Salt and pepper to taste
- 1 avocado, sliced
- Salsa (no added salt) for topping
- Fresh cilantro for garnish

Directions:
1. Heat the black beans with cumin, chili powder, salt, and pepper in a small saucepan until warmed through.
2. Warm the tortillas in a dry skillet or microwave.
3. Assemble the tacos by evenly layering the warmed black beans, avocado slices, and salsa on each tortilla.
4. Garnish the tacos with fresh cilantro before serving.

Per serving: Calories: 400kcal; Saturated fat: 2g; Sugar: 2g; Sodium: 350mg

23. Oat Bran Cereal with Almond Milk

Preparation time: 5 minutes

Cooking time: 5 minutes

Servings: 2

Ingredients:

- 1 cup oat bran
- 2 cups unsweetened almond milk
- 1/4 cup fresh berries (optional)
- 1 tablespoon chopped nuts (e.g., almonds, walnuts)
- 1 teaspoon honey or maple syrup (optional)

Directions:
1. Bring the almond milk to a gentle boil in a saucepan.
2. Stir in the oat bran, then reduce the heat to low.
3. Cook for 3-5 minutes, stirring frequently, until the oat bran thickens.
4. Remove the saucepan from the heat and let it sit for a minute.
5. Pour the cooked oat bran into bowls and top with fresh berries and chopped nuts.
6. Drizzle with honey or maple syrup if desired.

Per serving: Calories: 200kcal; Saturated fat: 0.5g; Sugar: 4g; Sodium: 150mg

24. Almond and Date Breakfast Bars

Preparation time: 15 minutes
Cooking time: 20 minutes
Servings: 8
Ingredients:

- 1 cup rolled oats
- 1/2 cup almond flour
- 1/4 cup shredded coconut
- 1/2 cup almonds, chopped
- 1/2 cup dates, pitted and chopped
- 1/4 cup almond butter
- 1/4 cup honey
- 1/4 cup unsweetened applesauce
- 1 teaspoon vanilla extract
- 1/4 teaspoon salt

Directions:
1. Preheat the oven to 350°F and line a baking dish with parchment paper.
2. In a large bowl, mix together the oats, almond flour, shredded coconut, chopped almonds, and dates.
3. Warm the almond butter, honey, applesauce, vanilla extract, and salt in a small saucepan until well combined.
4. Pour the wet ingredients over the dry ingredients and mix until everything is evenly coated.
5. Press the mixture into the prepared baking dish, ensuring it is evenly spread out.
6. Bake for 20 minutes, or until the edges are golden brown.
7. Let the mixture cool completely before cutting it into bars.

Per serving: Calories: 250kcal; Saturated fat: 2g; Sugar: 12g; Sodium: 50mg

25. Quinoa and Spinach Breakfast Casserole

Preparation time: 15 minutes
Cooking time: 30 minutes
Servings: 4
Ingredients:

- 1 cup quinoa, cooked
- 1 cup spinach, chopped
- 1/2 cup feta cheese, crumbled
- 4 large eggs
- 1 cup milk (unsweetened)
- 1 teaspoon dried oregano

- Salt and pepper to taste
- Cooking spray

Directions:
1. Preheat the oven to 375°F and coat a baking dish with cooking spray.
2. In a large bowl, mix together the cooked quinoa, chopped spinach, and crumbled feta cheese.
3. In another bowl, whisk the eggs, milk, oregano, salt, and pepper together.
4. Combine the wet and dry ingredients, then pour the mixture into the prepared baking dish.
5. Bake for 25-30 minutes, or until the eggs are set and the top of the casserole is golden brown.
6. Let the casserole cool slightly before serving.

Per serving: Calories: 300kcal; Saturated fat: 5g; Sugar: 2g; Sodium: 350mg

Snip Tasty Morsels: Healthy Snacks for Every Craving

26. Roasted Red Pepper Hummus with Carrot Sticks

Preparation time: 10 minutes

Cooking time: 0 minutes

Servings: 4

Ingredients:

- 1 can (15 oz) chickpeas, that is drained and rinsed
- 1 large red bell pepper, that is roasted and peeled
- 2 cloves garlic, minced
- 2 tablespoons tahini
- 2 tablespoons olive oil
- Juice of 1 lemon
- Carrot sticks for dipping

Directions:

1. Combine the chickpeas, roasted red pepper, minced garlic, tahini, olive oil, and lemon juice in a food processor.
2. Blend until smooth, scraping down the sides of the food processor as needed.
3. Serve the hummus with carrot sticks for a delicious and nutritious snack.

Per serving: Calories: 180kcal; Saturated fat: 1g; Sugar: 3g; Sodium: 210mg

27. Pear Slices with Cottage Cheese

Preparation time: 5 minutes

Cooking time: 0 minutes

Servings: 2

Ingredients:

- 1 ripe pear, sliced
- 1 cup low-fat cottage cheese

Directions:

1. Arrange the pear slices neatly on a plate.
2. Serve the pear slices with a side of low-fat cottage cheese.

Per serving: Calories: 200kcal; Saturated fat: 1.5g; Sugar: 9g; Sodium: 300mg

28. Baked Kale Chips

Preparation time: 10 minutes

Cooking time: 15 minutes

Servings: 2

Ingredients:

- 1 bunch kale, that is stems removed and leaves torn into bite-sized pieces
- 1 tablespoon olive oil
- Optional: Dash of lemon juice

Directions:

1. Preheat the oven to 350°F.
2. Toss the kale pieces with olive oil and, if desired, a dash of lemon juice in a bowl.
3. Spread the kale pieces in a single layer on a baking sheet.
4. Bake for 12-15 minutes, or until the kale chips are crisp but not burnt. Keep an eye on them to prevent burning.

Per serving: Calories: 120kcal; Saturated fat: 1g; Sugar: 1g; Sodium: 20mg

29. Cherry Tomato and Mozzarella Skewers

Preparation time: 10 minutes

Cooking time: 0 minutes

Servings: 4

Ingredients:

- 1 pint cherry tomatoes
- 1 cup mini mozzarella balls
- Fresh basil leaves
- Balsamic glaze (optional)

Directions:

1. Thread a cherry tomato, a mini mozzarella ball, and a basil leaf onto each small skewer.
2. Arrange skewers on a serving platter.
3. If desired, lightly drizzle the skewers with balsamic glaze before serving.

Per serving: Calories: 90kcal; Saturated fat: 3g; Sugar: 2g; Sodium: 30mg

30. Rice Cakes with Peanut Butter and Banana

Preparation time: 5 minutes

Cooking time: 0 minutes

Servings: 2

Ingredients:

- 2 rice cakes
- 2 tablespoons natural peanut butter
- 1 banana, sliced

Directions:
1. Spread the peanut butter evenly over the surface of each rice cake.
2. Arrange the banana slices on top of each rice cake, covering the peanut butter layer.

Per serving: Calories: 220kcal; Saturated fat: 1g; Sugar: 7g; Sodium: 80mg

31. Greek Yogurt with Pomegranate Seeds

Preparation time: 5 minutes

Cooking time: 0 minutes

Servings: 2

Ingredients:

- 1 cup plain Greek yogurt
- 1/2 cup pomegranate seeds

Directions:
1. Distribute the Greek yogurt evenly into two serving bowls.
2. Sprinkle the pomegranate seeds over the yogurt in each bowl.

Per serving: Calories: 150kcal; Saturated fat: 0g; Sugar: 8g; Sodium: 60mg

32. Mixed Nuts (Unsalted) and Sliced Apple

Preparation time: 5 minutes

Cooking time: 0 minutes

Servings: 2

Ingredients:

- 1 cup mixed nuts (almonds, walnuts, cashews) - unsalted
- 1 apple, sliced

Directions:
1. Arrange the mixed nuts evenly on a plate.
2. Serve the mixed nuts alongside the sliced apples for a satisfying and crunchy snack.

Per serving: Calories: 280kcal; Saturated fat: 3g; Sugar: 10g; Sodium: 5mg

33. Cucumber Slices with Greek Yogurt Dip

Preparation time: 10 minutes

Cooking time: 0 minutes

Servings: 4

Ingredients:

- 2 cucumbers, sliced
- 1 cup Greek yogurt
- 1 tablespoon fresh dill, chopped
- 1 clove garlic, minced
- Salt and pepper to taste

Directions:

1. In a small bowl, mix together the Greek yogurt, fresh dill, minced garlic, salt, and pepper.
2. Serve the cucumber slices alongside the Greek yogurt dip for dipping.

Per serving: Calories: 50kcal; Saturated fat: 0g; Sugar: 3g; Sodium: 20mg

34. Air-Popped Popcorn

Preparation time: 5 minutes

Cooking time: 5 minutes

Servings: 4

Ingredients:

- 1/2 cup popcorn kernels

Directions:

1. Air-pop the popcorn according to the manufacturer's instructions.
2. If desired, season the popcorn with a dash of your favorite herbs or spices for added flavor.

Per serving: Calories: 30kcal; Saturated fat: 0g; Sugar: 0g; Sodium: 0mg

35. Edamame

Preparation time: 5 minutes

Cooking time: 5 minutes

Servings: 2

Ingredients:

- 2 cups edamame (in pods)

Directions:

1. Steam the edamame in pods according to the package instructions.
2. Allow the steamed edamame to cool slightly before serving.

Per serving: Calories: 120kcal; Saturated fat: 0.5g; Sugar: 3g; Sodium: 5mg

36. Roasted Chickpeas

Preparation time: 10 minutes

Cooking time: 25 minutes

Servings: 4

Ingredients:

- 2 cans (15 oz each) chickpeas, that is drained and rinsed
- 2 tablespoons olive oil
- 1 teaspoon cumin
- 1 teaspoon paprika
- 1/2 teaspoon garlic powder

Directions:

1. Preheat the oven to 400°F.
2. Toss the chickpeas with olive oil, cumin, paprika, and garlic powder in a bowl until evenly coated.
3. Spread the chickpeas in a single layer on a baking sheet and roast for 25 minutes, or until they are crispy.

Per serving: Calories: 180kcal; Saturated fat: 1g; Sugar: 2g; Sodium: 10mg

37. Sliced Bell Peppers with Guacamole

Preparation time: 10 minutes

Cooking time: 0 minutes

Servings: 4

Ingredients:

- 2 bell peppers (any color), sliced
- 2 avocados, mashed
- 1 tomato, diced
- 1/4 cup red onion, finely chopped
- 1 clove garlic, minced
- Juice of 1 lime
- Salt and pepper to taste

Directions:

1. Arrange the bell pepper slices neatly on a serving plate.
2. In a bowl, mix together the mashed avocados, diced tomato, finely chopped red onion, minced garlic, lime juice, salt, and pepper to make guacamole.
3. Serve the bell pepper slices alongside the guacamole for dipping.

Per serving: Calories: 150kcal; Saturated fat: 2g; Sugar: 3g; Sodium: 10mg

38. Watermelon Cubes

Preparation time: 10 minutes
Cooking time: 0 minutes
Servings: 4
Ingredients:

- 1 small watermelon, cut into cubes

Directions:
1. Carefully remove the seeds from the watermelon and cut the flesh into bite-sized cubes.

Per serving: Calories: 45kcal; Saturated fat: 0g; Sugar: 9g; Sodium: 0mg

39. Pineapple and Cottage Cheese

Preparation time: 5 minutes
Cooking time: 0 minutes
Servings: 2
Ingredients:

- 1 cup pineapple chunks (fresh or canned, in juice)
- 1/2 cup low-fat cottage cheese

Directions:
1. In a bowl, gently mix together the pineapple chunks and low-fat cottage cheese.
2. Serve immediately.

Per serving: Calories: 120kcal; Saturated fat: 1g; Sugar: 14g; Sodium: 300mg

40. Almond Butter and Banana Slices

Preparation time: 5 minutes
Cooking time: 0 minutes
Servings: 2
Ingredients:

- 2 tablespoons almond butter (unsweetened)
- 1 banana, sliced

Directions:
1. Spread the almond butter evenly over the banana slice.
2. Enjoy this simple and satisfying snack.

Per serving: Calories: 220kcal; Saturated fat: 1.5g; Sugar: 12g; Sodium: 5mg

41. Greek Yogurt with Papaya

Preparation time: 5 minutes

Cooking time: 0 minutes

Servings: 2

Ingredients:

- 1 cup plain Greek yogurt
- 1 cup ripe papaya, diced

Directions:

1. Distribute the Greek yogurt evenly into two serving bowls.
2. Top each bowl of yogurt with the diced papaya.

Per serving: Calories: 180kcal; Saturated fat: 0g; Sugar: 15g; Sodium: 70mg

42. Sliced Mango with Lime

Preparation time: 5 minutes

Cooking time: 0 minutes

Servings: 2

Ingredients:

- 2 ripe mangoes, sliced
- 1 lime, juiced

Directions:

1. Arrange the mango slices neatly on a serving plate.
2. Drizzle the freshly squeezed lime juice evenly over the mango slices.

Per serving: Calories: 120kcal; Saturated fat: 0g; Sugar: 28g; Sodium: 0mg

43. Celery Sticks with Hummus and Raisins

Preparation time: 10 minutes

Cooking time: 0 minutes

Servings: 2

Ingredients:

- 4 celery stalks, cut into sticks
- 1/2 cup hummus
- 2 tablespoons raisins

Directions:

1. Spread the hummus evenly over each celery stick.
2. Sprinkle the raisins over the hummus-covered celery sticks to add a sweet and savory crunch.

Per serving: Calories: 180kcal; Saturated fat: 1g; Sugar: 6g; Sodium: 320mg

44. Mixed Berries with Greek Yogurt

Preparation time: 5 minutes
Cooking time: 0 minutes
Servings: 2
Ingredients:

- 1 cup mixed berries (strawberries, blueberries, raspberries)
- 1 cup plain Greek yogurt

Directions:
1. Distribute the Greek yogurt evenly between two serving bowls.
2. Top each bowl of yogurt with an assortment of mixed berries.

Per serving: Calories: 150kcal; Saturated fat: 0g; Sugar: 12g; Sodium: 40mg

45. Apple Cinnamon Rice Cakes

Preparation time: 5 minutes
Cooking time: 0 minutes
Servings: 2
Ingredients:

- 2 rice cakes
- 1 medium apple, thinly sliced
- 1 teaspoon ground cinnamon

Directions:
1. Arrange the thinly sliced apple pieces evenly on each rice cake.
2. Lightly sprinkle ground cinnamon over the apple slices on each rice cake.

Per serving: Calories: 90kcal; Saturated fat: 0g; Sugar: 8g; Sodium: 0mg

Bowls of Bounty: Heartwarming Soups & Crisp Salads

46. Quinoa and Black Bean Salad

Preparation time: 15 minutes
Cooking time: 15 minutes
Servings: 4
Ingredients:

- 1 cup quinoa, rinsed
- 2 cups water
- 1 can (15 oz) black beans, that is drained and rinsed
- 1 cup cherry tomatoes, halved
- 1 cucumber, diced
- 1/4 cup red onion, finely chopped
- 2 tablespoons olive oil
- 2 tablespoons fresh lime juice
- Salt-free cumin (to taste)
- Salt-free chili powder (to taste)
- Fresh cilantro, chopped (optional)

Directions:

1. Cook quinoa according to package instructions.
2. In a large bowl, combine the cooked quinoa, black beans, halved cherry tomatoes, diced cucumber, and finely chopped red onion.
3. In a small bowl, whisk together the olive oil, fresh lime juice, salt-free cumin, and chili powder.
4. Pour the dressing over the salad and toss gently to ensure all ingredients are evenly coated.
5. Garnish with chopped fresh cilantro if desired.
6. Serve chilled.

Per serving: Calories: 320kcal; Saturated fat: 1g; Sugar: 4g; Sodium: 20mg

47. Roasted Beet and Goat Cheese Salad

Preparation time: 10 minutes
Cooking time: 40 minutes (for roasting beets)
Servings: 4
Ingredients:

- 4 medium-sized beets, peeled and diced
- 2 tablespoons olive oil
- Salt-free black pepper (to taste)
- 4 cups mixed salad greens
- 1/2 cup crumbled goat cheese
- 1/4 cup balsamic vinegar
- 1 tablespoon Dijon mustard

Directions:

1. Preheat the oven to 400°F.
2. Toss the diced beets with olive oil and a sprinkle of salt-free black pepper, then spread them out evenly on a baking sheet.
3. Roast the beets for 40 minutes, or until they are tender, stirring occasionally.
4. In a large bowl, combine the roasted beets, mixed salad greens, and crumbled goat cheese.
5. In a small bowl, whisk together the balsamic vinegar and Dijon mustard.
6. Drizzle the dressing over the salad and toss gently to combine.
7. Serve immediately.

Per serving: Calories: 180kcal; Saturated fat: 2g; Sugar: 8g; Sodium: 40mg

48. Spinach and Chickpea Salad with Lemon Vinaigrette

Preparation time: 15 minutes
Cooking time: 0 minutes
Servings: 4
Ingredients:

- 6 cups fresh spinach leaves
- 1 can (15 oz) chickpeas, that is drained and rinsed
- 1 cup cherry tomatoes, halved
- 1/4 cup red onion, thinly sliced
- 1/3 cup feta cheese, crumbled
- 2 tablespoons olive oil
- 2 tablespoons fresh lemon juice
- Salt-free garlic powder (to taste)
- Salt-free black pepper (to taste)

Directions:
1. In a large bowl, combine the spinach leaves, chickpeas, halved cherry tomatoes, thinly sliced red onion, and crumbled feta cheese.
2. In a small bowl, whisk together the olive oil, fresh lemon juice, salt-free garlic powder, and salt-free black pepper.
3. Drizzle the dressing over the salad and toss gently to ensure all the ingredients are evenly coated.
4. Serve immediately.

Per serving: Calories: 250kcal; Saturated fat: 2g; Sugar: 3g; Sodium: 60mg

49. Mushroom Barley Soup

Preparation time: 15 minutes
Cooking time: 45 minutes
Servings: 6
Ingredients:

- 1 cup pearl barley, rinsed
- 8 cups low-sodium vegetable broth
- 2 cups mushrooms, sliced
- 1 onion, diced
- 2 carrots, diced
- 2 celery stalks, diced
- 2 cloves garlic, minced
- 1 teaspoon dried thyme
- Salt-free black pepper (to taste)
- Fresh parsley, chopped (for garnish)

Directions:
1. In a large pot, combine the pearl barley and low-sodium vegetable broth. Bring it to a boil, then reduce the heat to simmer for 30 minutes.
2. In a separate pan, sauté the sliced mushrooms, diced onion, diced carrots, diced celery, and minced garlic until they are softened.
3. Add the sautéed vegetables to the pot containing the barley.
4. Season the soup with dried thyme and salt-free black pepper, and continue to simmer for an additional 15 minutes.
5. Garnish the soup with chopped fresh parsley before serving.

Per serving: Calories: 180kcal; Saturated fat: 0.2g; Sugar: 2g; Sodium: 30mg

50. Greek Quinoa Salad

Preparation time: 15 minutes

Cooking time: 15 minutes

Servings: 4

Ingredients:

- 1 cup quinoa, rinsed
- 2 cups water
- 1 cucumber, diced
- 1 cup cherry tomatoes, halved
- 1/2 cup Kalamata olives, sliced
- 1/2 cup feta cheese, crumbled
- 1/4 cup red onion, finely chopped
- 3 tablespoons olive oil
- 2 tablespoons red wine vinegar
- Salt-free oregano (to taste)
- Salt-free black pepper (to taste)

Directions:

1. Cook quinoa according to package instructions.
2. In a large bowl, combine the crumbled feta cheese, cooked quinoa, diced cucumber, halved cherry tomatoes, sliced olives, and finely chopped red onion.
3. In a small bowl, whisk together the olive oil, red wine vinegar, salt-free oregano, and salt-free black pepper.
4. Pour the dressing over the salad and toss gently to ensure all ingredients are evenly coated.
5. Serve chilled.

Per serving: Calories: 350kcal; Saturated fat: 2g; Sugar: 4g; Sodium: 90mg

51. Roasted Butternut Squash Salad

Preparation time: 20 minutes

Cooking time: 25 minutes

Servings: 4

Ingredients:

- 4 cups butternut squash, peeled and cubed
- 2 tablespoons olive oil
- Salt-free black pepper (to taste)
- 6 cups mixed salad greens
- 1/2 cup dried cranberries
- 1/4 cup pumpkin seeds

- 1/4 cup balsamic vinegar
- 1 tablespoon maple syrup (optional)

Directions:
1. Preheat the oven to 400°F.
2. Toss the cubed butternut squash with olive oil and a sprinkle of salt-free black pepper, then spread it out evenly on a baking sheet.
3. Roast the butternut squash for 25 minutes, or until it is tender, stirring occasionally.
4. In a large bowl, combine the roasted butternut squash, mixed salad greens, dried cranberries, and pumpkin seeds.
5. In a small bowl, whisk together the balsamic vinegar and maple syrup (if using).
6. Drizzle the dressing over the salad and toss gently to combine.
7. Serve immediately.

Per serving: Calories: 250kcal; Saturated fat: 1g; Sugar: 12g; Sodium: 20mg

52. Chicken and Vegetable Stir-Fry Soup

Preparation time: 15 minutes

Cooking time: 20 minutes

Servings: 4

Ingredients:
- 1 lb boneless, that is skinless chicken breast, thinly sliced
- 1 tablespoon low-sodium soy sauce
- 1 tablespoon sesame oil
- 2 cloves garlic, minced
- 1 teaspoon ginger, grated
- 4 cups low-sodium chicken broth
- 2 cups broccoli florets
- 1 bell pepper, thinly sliced
- 1 carrot, julienned
- 1 cup snap peas, ends trimmed
- 1 cup cabbage, shredded
- Green onions, chopped (for garnish)

Directions:
1. In a bowl, marinate the thinly sliced chicken in low-sodium soy sauce and sesame oil.
2. In a large pot, sauté the minced garlic and grated ginger until fragrant.
3. Add the marinated chicken to the pot and cook until browned.
4. Pour in the low-sodium chicken broth and bring to a simmer.
5. Add the broccoli florets, thinly sliced bell pepper, julienned carrot, trimmed snap peas, and shredded cabbage. Simmer for 10-15 minutes until the vegetables are tender.

6. Garnish the soup with chopped green onions before serving.

Per serving: Calories: 220kcal; Saturated fat: 0.8g; Sugar: 4g; Sodium: 50mg

53. Spinach and Pomegranate Salad

Preparation time: 10 minutes
Cooking time: 0 minutes
Servings: 4
Ingredients:

- 6 cups fresh spinach leaves
- 1 cup pomegranate seeds
- 1/2 cup walnuts, chopped
- 1/4 cup feta cheese, crumbled
- 2 tablespoons olive oil
- 1 tablespoon balsamic vinegar
- Salt-free black pepper (to taste)

Directions:

1. In a large bowl, combine the fresh spinach leaves, pomegranate seeds, chopped walnuts, and crumbled feta cheese.
2. In a small bowl, whisk together the olive oil, balsamic vinegar, and a sprinkle of salt-free black pepper.
3. Drizzle the dressing over the salad and toss gently to coat evenly.
4. Serve immediately.

Per serving: Calories: 240kcal; Saturated fat: 2g; Sugar: 8g; Sodium: 30mg

54. Lentil and Vegetable Soup

Preparation time: 15 minutes
Cooking time: 40 minutes
Servings: 6
Ingredients:

- 1 cup dried green lentils, rinsed
- 8 cups low-sodium vegetable broth
- 1 onion, chopped
- 2 carrots, diced
- 2 celery stalks, diced
- 2 cloves garlic, minced
- 1 teaspoon cumin
- 1 teaspoon paprika
- Salt-free black pepper (to taste)

- Fresh parsley, chopped (for garnish)

Directions:
1. In a large pot, combine the rinsed green lentils and low-sodium vegetable broth. Bring to a boil, then reduce the heat and simmer for 25-30 minutes.
2. In a separate pan, sauté the chopped onions, diced carrots, diced celery, and minced garlic until they are softened.
3. Add the sautéed vegetables to the pot containing the lentils.
4. Season the soup with cumin, paprika, and salt-free black pepper, and continue to simmer for an additional 10-15 minutes.
5. Garnish the soup with chopped fresh parsley before serving.

Per serving: Calories: 180kcal; Saturated fat: 0.2g; Sugar: 4g; Sodium: 40mg

55. Caprese Salad with Balsamic Glaze

Preparation time: 10 minutes
Cooking time: 0 minutes
Servings: 4
Ingredients:

- 2 cups cherry tomatoes, halved
- 1 cup fresh mozzarella cheese, diced
- Fresh basil leaves, torn
- 2 tablespoons balsamic glaze
- 1 tablespoon olive oil
- Salt-free black pepper (to taste)

Directions:
1. In a bowl, combine the halved cherry tomatoes, diced fresh mozzarella, and torn basil leaves.
2. Drizzle the salad with balsamic glaze and olive oil.
3. Season with salt-free black pepper to taste and toss gently to combine the ingredients.
4. Serve immediately.

Per serving: Calories: 180kcal; Saturated fat: 2g; Sugar: 3g; Sodium: 60mg

56. Avocado and Quinoa Salad

Preparation time: 15 minutes
Cooking time: 15 minutes
Servings: 4
Ingredients:

- 1 cup quinoa, rinsed
- 2 cups water

- 2 ripe avocados, diced
- 1 cup cherry tomatoes, halved
- 1/4 cup red onion, finely chopped
- 1/4 cup fresh cilantro, chopped
- 2 tablespoons olive oil
- 2 tablespoons lime juice
- Salt-free cumin (to taste)
- Salt-free black pepper (to taste)

Directions:
1. Cook quinoa according to package instructions.
2. In a large bowl, combine the cooked quinoa, diced avocados, halved cherry tomatoes, finely chopped red onion, and chopped cilantro.
3. In a small bowl, whisk together the olive oil, lime juice, salt-free cumin, and salt-free black pepper.
4. Pour the dressing over the salad and toss gently to ensure all ingredients are evenly coated.
5. Serve chilled.

Per serving: Calories: 320kcal; Saturated fat: 2g; Sugar: 2g; Sodium: 10mg

57. Kale and Cranberry Salad

Preparation time: 15 minutes
Cooking time: 0 minutes
Servings: 4
Ingredients:

- 6 cups kale, that is stems removed, and leaves chopped
- 1/2 cup dried cranberries
- 1/4 cup sunflower seeds
- 1/4 cup feta cheese, crumbled
- 3 tablespoons olive oil
- 2 tablespoons balsamic vinegar
- Salt-free black pepper (to taste)

Directions:
1. In a large bowl, combine the chopped kale, dried cranberries, sunflower seeds, and crumbled feta cheese.
2. In a small bowl, whisk together the olive oil, balsamic vinegar, and a sprinkle of salt-free black pepper.
3. Drizzle the dressing over the salad and toss gently to coat all the ingredients evenly.
4. Serve immediately.

Per serving: Calories: 250kcal; Saturated fat: 2g; Sugar: 6g; Sodium: 30mg

58. Tomato Cucumber Salad with Dill

Preparation time: 10 minutes
Cooking time: 0 minutes
Servings: 4
Ingredients:

- 2 cups cherry tomatoes, halved
- 1 cucumber, sliced
- 1/4 cup red onion, thinly sliced
- 2 tablespoons fresh dill, chopped
- 2 tablespoons olive oil
- 1 tablespoon red wine vinegar
- Salt-free black pepper (to taste)

Directions:

1. In a bowl, combine the halved cherry tomatoes, sliced cucumber, thinly sliced red onion, and chopped fresh dill.
2. In a small bowl, whisk together the olive oil, red wine vinegar, and a sprinkle of salt-free black pepper.
3. Pour the dressing over the salad and toss gently to ensure all the ingredients are evenly coated.
4. Serve immediately.

Per serving: Calories: 120kcal; Saturated fat: 1g; Sugar: 3g; Sodium: 10mg

59. Gazpacho with Cucumber Salsa

Preparation time: 15 minutes
Cooking time: 0 minutes
Servings: 4
Ingredients:

- 6 large tomatoes, chopped
- 1 cucumber, peeled and chopped
- 1 bell pepper (any color), chopped
- 1/4 cup red onion, chopped
- 2 cloves garlic, minced
- 3 cups tomato juice
- 1/4 cup red wine vinegar
- 2 tablespoons olive oil
- Salt-free black pepper (to taste)
- 1/2 cup cucumber, diced (for salsa)

Directions:
1. In a blender, combine the chopped tomatoes, peeled and chopped cucumber, chopped bell pepper, chopped red onion, minced garlic, tomato juice, red wine vinegar, and olive oil. Blend until smooth.
2. Season the gazpacho with salt-free black pepper to taste.
3. Refrigerate the gazpacho for at least 2 hours before serving to allow the flavors to meld.
4. Prepare the cucumber salsa by combining the diced cucumber with a pinch of salt and pepper in a separate bowl.
5. Serve the chilled Gazpacho, topped with the cucumber salsa.

Per serving: Calories: 150kcal; Saturated fat: 1g; Sugar: 8g; Sodium: 20mg

60. Roasted Garlic and White Bean Soup

Preparation time: 10 minutes
Cooking time: 30 minutes
Servings: 4
Ingredients:

- 2 cans (15 oz each) white beans, that is drained and rinsed
- 4 cups low-sodium vegetable broth
- 1 head garlic, roasted
- 1 onion, chopped
- 2 carrots, chopped
- 2 celery stalks, chopped
- 2 tablespoons olive oil
- 1 teaspoon thyme, dried
- Salt-free black pepper (to taste)

Directions:
1. Roast the garlic by cutting off the top of the head, drizzling it with olive oil, wrapping it in foil, and then baking it at 400°F for 30 minutes.
2. In a large pot, sauté the chopped onion, carrots, and celery in olive oil until they are softened.
3. Add the drained and rinsed white beans, low-sodium vegetable broth, roasted garlic cloves (squeezed out of their skins), and dried thyme. Simmer the soup for 15-20 minutes.
4. Use an immersion blender to blend the soup until smooth, or carefully transfer it to a blender to puree.
5. Season the soup with salt-free black pepper to taste.
6. Serve hot.

Per serving: Calories: 250kcal; Saturated fat: 1g; Sugar: 3g; Sodium: 50mg

Prime Plates: Meaty Mains with a Healthy Twist

61. Grilled Lemon Herb Chicken

Preparation time: 10 minutes
Cooking time: 15 minutes
Servings: 4
Ingredients:

- 4 boneless, skinless chicken breasts
- 2 tablespoons olive oil
- 1 lemon (juiced)
- 2 cloves garlic (minced)
- 1 teaspoon dried oregano
- 1 teaspoon dried thyme
- Salt and pepper to taste

Directions:

1. Preheat your grill to medium-high heat.
2. In a small bowl, mix together the olive oil, lemon juice, minced garlic, dried oregano, dried thyme, salt, and pepper to create a marinade.
3. Place the chicken breasts in a shallow dish and coat them evenly with the marinade.
4. Grill the chicken for 6-8 minutes per side, or until it is fully cooked and reaches an internal temperature of 165°F.
5. Serve hot, and enjoy!

Per serving: Calories: 220kcal; Saturated fat: 2g; Sugar: 0g; Sodium: 80mg

62. Turkey and Spinach Stuffed Mushrooms

Preparation time: 15 minutes
Cooking time: 20 minutes
Servings: 6
Ingredients:

- 24 large button mushrooms, that is cleaned and stems removed
- 1/2 pound lean ground turkey
- 1 cup fresh spinach, chopped
- 1/2 onion, finely diced
- 2 cloves garlic, minced
- 1 teaspoon olive oil

- Salt and pepper to taste
- 1/4 cup grated Parmesan cheese

Directions:
1. Preheat the oven to 375°F.
2. In a skillet, heat the olive oil over medium heat. Add the onions and garlic, sautéing until they are softened.
3. Add the ground turkey to the skillet and cook until browned. Then add the chopped spinach and cook until it wilts. Season with salt and pepper to taste.
4. Spoon the turkey and spinach mixture into each mushroom cap, arranging them on a baking sheet.
5. Sprinkle Parmesan cheese over the stuffed mushrooms, then bake for 15-20 minutes, or until the mushrooms are tender.

Per serving: Calories: 120kcal; Saturated fat: 1g; Sugar: 2g; Sodium: 70mg

63. Beef and Broccoli Stir-Fry

Preparation time: 15 minutes
Cooking time: 10 minutes
Servings: 4
Ingredients:

- 1 pound lean beef strips (such as sirloin or flank steak)
- 4 cups broccoli florets
- 3 tablespoons low-sodium soy sauce
- 1 tablespoon honey
- 2 cloves garlic, minced
- 1 teaspoon ginger, grated
- 2 tablespoons vegetable oil
- Sesame seeds for garnish (optional)

Directions:
1. In a small bowl, mix together the low-sodium soy sauce, honey, minced garlic, and grated ginger to create the sauce.
2. Heat the vegetable oil in a large skillet over medium-high heat.
3. Add the beef strips to the skillet and cook until browned, removing any excess liquid if necessary.
4. Add the broccoli florets to the skillet and stir-fry for 3-4 minutes until they are tender-crisp.
5. Pour the sauce over the beef and broccoli in the skillet, tossing everything together to coat evenly.
6. Cook for an additional 2-3 minutes until the sauce has thickened.
7. Garnish with sesame seeds if desired, and serve the stir-fry hot.

Per serving: Calories: 280kcal; Saturated fat: 2g; Sugar: 6g; Sodium: 400mg

64. Pork Tenderloin with Mustard Sauce

Preparation time: 10 minutes

Cooking time: 25 minutes

Servings: 4

Ingredients:

- 1 pound pork tenderloin
- Salt and pepper to taste
- 1 tablespoon olive oil
- 2 tablespoons Dijon mustard
- 1 tablespoon honey
- 1 clove garlic, minced
- 1/2 cup low-sodium chicken broth

Directions:

1. Preheat the oven to 375°F.
2. Season the pork tenderloin generously with salt and pepper.
3. In an oven-safe skillet, heat the olive oil over medium-high heat.
4. Sear the pork on all sides until it is well browned.
5. In a small bowl, whisk together the Dijon mustard, honey, minced garlic, and low-sodium chicken broth.
6. Pour the mustard sauce over the seared pork in the skillet.
7. Transfer the skillet to the preheated oven and roast for 20-25 minutes, or until the internal temperature of the pork reaches 145°F.
8. Allow the pork tenderloin to rest for a few minutes before slicing and serving to ensure the juices redistribute.

Per serving: Calories: 220kcal; Saturated fat: 2g; Sugar: 4g; Sodium: 180mg

65. Chicken and Veggie Skewers with Tzatziki

Preparation time: 20 minutes

Cooking time: 15 minutes

Servings: 4

Ingredients:

- 1 pound boneless, skinless chicken breast, cut into chunks
- 1 bell pepper, cut into chunks
- 1 zucchini, sliced
- 1 red onion, cut into chunks
- 2 tablespoons olive oil
- 1 teaspoon dried oregano

- Salt and pepper to taste
- For Tzatziki:
- 1 cup Greek yogurt
- 1/2 cucumber, finely diced
- 1 clove garlic, minced
- 1 tablespoon fresh dill, chopped
- Salt and pepper to taste

Directions:
1. Preheat the grill or oven broiler.
2. In a large bowl, combine the chicken chunks, chunks of bell pepper, sliced zucchini, chunks of red onion, olive oil, dried oregano, salt, and pepper.
3. Thread the marinated chicken and vegetables onto skewers, alternating pieces for variety.
4. Grill or broil the skewers for 10-15 minutes, turning them occasionally, until the chicken is fully cooked and the vegetables are tender.
5. For the Tzatziki sauce, in a separate bowl, mix together the Greek yogurt, finely diced cucumber, minced garlic, chopped fresh dill, salt, and pepper.
6. Serve the skewers with Tzatziki on the side.

Per serving: Calories: 280kcal; Saturated fat: 2g; Sugar: 4g; Sodium: 120mg

66. Baked Turkey Meatloaf

Preparation time: 15 minutes
Cooking time: 45 minutes
Servings: 6
Ingredients:

- 1.5 pounds ground turkey
- 1 cup whole wheat breadcrumbs
- 1/2 cup skim milk
- 1 egg
- 1/2 onion, finely diced
- 1 carrot, grated
- 1/2 cup ketchup (no added sugar)
- 1 teaspoon Worcestershire sauce
- Salt and pepper to taste

Directions:
1. Preheat the oven to 375°F.
2. In a large bowl, combine the ground turkey, whole wheat breadcrumbs, skim milk, egg, finely diced onion, grated carrot, ketchup, Worcestershire sauce, salt, and pepper. Mix until all the ingredients are well combined.

3. Transfer the mixture into a lightly greased loaf pan, and shape it into a loaf.
4. Bake for 40-45 minutes, or until the meatloaf's internal temperature reaches 165°F, indicating it is fully cooked.
5. Allow the meatloaf to rest for a few minutes before slicing to ensure it retains its juices.

Per serving: Calories: 250kcal; Saturated fat: 2g; Sugar: 5g; Sodium: 350mg

67. Beef and Vegetable Stir-Fry

Preparation time: 15 minutes
Cooking time: 10 minutes
Servings: 4
Ingredients:

- 1 pound lean beef strips (such as sirloin or flank steak)
- 3 cups mixed vegetables (broccoli, bell peppers, snap peas)
- 2 tablespoons low-sodium soy sauce
- 1 tablespoon hoisin sauce
- 1 teaspoon sesame oil
- 2 cloves garlic, minced
- 1 teaspoon ginger, grated
- 2 tablespoons vegetable oil

Directions:
1. In a small bowl, mix together the low-sodium soy sauce, hoisin sauce, sesame oil, minced garlic, and grated ginger to create the sauce.
2. Heat the vegetable oil in a large skillet or wok over medium-high heat.
3. Add the beef strips to the skillet or wok and stir-fry until browned, removing any excess liquid if necessary.
4. Add the mixed vegetables to the skillet or wok and stir-fry for 3-4 minutes until they are tender-crisp.
5. Pour the sauce over the beef and vegetables, tossing everything together to coat evenly.
6. Continue to cook for an additional 2-3 minutes until the sauce has thickened.
7. Serve the stir-fry hot, ideally over a bed of rice or noodles if desired.

Per serving: Calories: 280kcal; Saturated fat: 2g; Sugar: 6g; Sodium: 420mg

68. Lemon Garlic Chicken Thighs

Preparation time: 10 minutes
Cooking time: 25 minutes
Servings: 4
Ingredients:

- 4 bone-in, skinless chicken thighs
- 2 tablespoons olive oil
- 2 lemons (juiced)
- 4 cloves garlic, minced
- 1 teaspoon dried thyme
- Salt and pepper to taste

Directions:

1. Preheat the oven to 400°F.
2. In a small bowl, mix together the olive oil, lemon juice, minced garlic, dried thyme, salt, and pepper to create the marinade.
3. Place the chicken thighs in a baking dish and coat them evenly with the lemon-garlic mixture.
4. Bake for 20-25 minutes, or until the chicken reaches an internal temperature of 165°F, ensuring it's fully cooked.
5. Spoon the juices from the baking dish over the chicken before serving to enhance the flavor.

Per serving: Calories: 280kcal; Saturated fat: 3g; Sugar: 2g; Sodium: 120mg

69. Pork Chops with Apple and Cabbage

Preparation time: 15 minutes
Cooking time: 25 minutes
Servings: 4
Ingredients:

- 4 boneless pork chops
- 2 apples, cored and sliced
- 1/2 head cabbage, thinly sliced
- 1 onion, thinly sliced
- 2 tablespoons olive oil
- 2 tablespoons apple cider vinegar
- 1 teaspoon caraway seeds
- Salt and pepper to taste

Directions:

1. Season the pork chops generously with salt and pepper on both sides.
2. Heat the olive oil in a large skillet over medium-high hea.

3. Add the pork chops to the skillet and sear them on both sides until browned, approximately 4-5 minutes per side.
4. Remove the pork chops from the skillet and set them aside on a plate.
5. In the same skillet, add the sliced apples, thinly sliced cabbage, and onion. Sauté for 5-7 minutes until they are softened.
6. Stir in the apple cider vinegar and caraway seeds, mixing well.
7. Return the pork chops to the skillet and cook for an additional 8-10 minutes, or until the pork reaches an internal temperature of 145°F, indicating it is cooked through.
8. Serve the pork chops over the sautéed apple and cabbage mixture, spooning any pan juices over the top.

Per serving: Calories: 320kcal; Saturated fat: 2g; Sugar: 10g; Sodium: 80mg

70. Teriyaki Chicken

Preparation time: 10 minutes
Cooking time: 15 minutes
Servings: 4
Ingredients:

- 1 pound boneless, that is skinless chicken breasts, cut into strips
- 2 cups broccoli florets
- 1 bell pepper, sliced
- 1/2 cup low-sodium teriyaki sauce
- 2 tablespoons low-sodium soy sauce
- 1 tablespoon honey
- 1 teaspoon sesame oil
- 2 cloves garlic, minced
- 1 teaspoon ginger, grated
- 2 tablespoons vegetable oil
- Sesame seeds for garnish (optional)

Directions:

1. In a small bowl, mix together the low-sodium teriyaki sauce, low-sodium soy sauce, honey, sesame oil, minced garlic, and grated ginger to create the sauce.
2. Heat the vegetable oil in a large skillet or wok over medium-high heat.
3. Add the chicken strips to the skillet or wok and stir-fry until they are browned and cooked through.
4. Add the broccoli florets and sliced bell pepper to the skillet, and continue stir-frying for another 3-4 minutes until the vegetables are tender-crisp.
5. Pour the sauce over the chicken and vegetables in the skillet, tossing everything together to coat evenly.
6. Continue to cook for an additional 2-3 minutes until the sauce has thickened.

7. Garnish with sesame seeds if desired, and serve the teriyaki chicken over brown rice for a complete mea.

Per serving: Calories: 280kcal; Saturated fat: 2g; Sugar: 8g; Sodium: 250mg

71. Lemon Dill Turkey Breast

Preparation time: 10 minutes

Cooking time: 35 minutes

Servings: 4

Ingredients:

- 1 pound turkey breast, boneless and skinless
- 2 tablespoons olive oil
- 1 lemon (juiced)
- 2 cloves garlic, minced
- 1 tablespoon fresh dill, chopped
- Salt and pepper to taste

Directions:

1. Preheat the oven to 375°F.
2. In a small bowl, mix together the olive oil, lemon juice, minced garlic, chopped fresh dill, salt, and pepper to create the marinade.
3. Place the turkey breast in a baking dish and evenly coat it with the lemon-dill marinade.
4. Bake for 30-35 minutes, or until the turkey breast reaches an internal temperature of 165°F, indicating it is fully cooked.
5. Allow the turkey breast to rest for a few minutes before slicing to ensure the juices redistribute throughout the meat.

Per serving: Calories: 220kcal; Saturated fat: 2g; Sugar: 1g; Sodium: 80mg

72. Beef and Pepper Stir-Fry

Preparation time: 15 minutes

Cooking time: 10 minutes

Servings: 4

Ingredients:

- 1 pound lean beef strips (such as sirloin or flank steak)
- 2 bell peppers, sliced
- 1 onion, thinly sliced
- 2 tablespoons low-sodium soy sauce
- 1 tablespoon hoisin sauce
- 1 teaspoon sesame oil
- 2 cloves garlic, minced

- 1 teaspoon ginger, grated
- 2 tablespoons vegetable oil

Directions:
1. In a small bowl, mix together the low-sodium soy sauce, hoisin sauce, sesame oil, minced garlic, and grated ginger to create the sauce.
2. Heat the vegetable oil in a large skillet or wok over medium-high heat.
3. Add the beef strips to the skillet or wok and stir-fry until they are browned, removing any excess liquid if necessary.
4. Add the sliced bell peppers and onion to the skillet or wok, and continue stir-frying for 3-4 minutes until they are tender-crisp.
5. Pour the sauce over the beef and vegetables in the skillet or wok, tossing everything together to coat evenly.
6. Continue to cook for an additional 2-3 minutes until the sauce has thickened.
7. Serve the stir-fry hot, ideally with a side of brown rice or noodles for a complete meal.

Per serving: Calories: 280kcal; Saturated fat: 2g; Sugar: 6g; Sodium: 420mg

73. Herb-Crusted Pork Tenderloin

Preparation time: 15 minutes
Cooking time: 25 minutes
Servings: 4
Ingredients:

- 1 pound pork tenderloin
- 2 tablespoons Dijon mustard
- 2 tablespoons fresh parsley, chopped
- 1 tablespoon fresh thyme, chopped
- 1 tablespoon fresh rosemary, chopped
- 2 cloves garlic, minced
- Salt and pepper to taste
- 1 tablespoon olive oil

Directions:
1. Preheat the oven to 400°F.
2. In a small bowl, mix together the Dijon mustard, chopped parsley, thyme, rosemary, minced garlic, salt, and pepper to create the herb crust mixture.
3. Pat the pork tenderloin dry with paper towels and then evenly rub the mustard-herb mixture over its entire surface.
4. Heat the olive oil in an oven-safe skillet over medium-high heat.
5. Sear the pork on all sides until it is well browned on each side.

6. Transfer the skillet to the preheated oven and roast for 20-25 minutes, or until the internal temperature of the pork reaches 145°F.
7. Allow the pork tenderloin to rest for a few minutes before slicing to ensure the juices redistribute throughout the meat.

Per serving: Calories: 250kcal; Saturated fat: 2g; Sugar: 0g; Sodium: 200mg

74. Turkey and Zucchini Meatballs

Preparation time: 15 minutes
Cooking time: 20 minutes
Servings: 4
Ingredients:

- 1 pound ground turkey
- 1 zucchini, that is grated and excess moisture squeezed out
- 1/2 cup whole wheat breadcrumbs
- 1/4 cup grated Parmesan cheese
- 1 egg
- 2 cloves garlic, minced
- 1 teaspoon dried oregano
- Salt and pepper to taste
- Marinara sauce for serving

Directions:

1. Preheat the oven to 375°F.
2. In a large bowl, combine the ground turkey, grated zucchini (with excess moisture squeezed out), whole wheat breadcrumbs, grated Parmesan cheese, egg, minced garlic, dried oregano, salt, and pepper. Mix until the ingredients are well combined.
3. Bake for 18-20 minutes, or until the meatballs are cooked through and reach an internal temperature of 165°F.
4. Bake for 18-20 minutes or 'til the meatballs are cooked through.
5. Heat the marinara sauce in a saucepan over medium heat and serve the baked meatballs with the sauce, either on top or on the side, as preferred.

Per serving: Calories: 230kcal; Saturated fat: 2g; Sugar: 2g; Sodium: 350mg

75. Lean Beef and Vegetable Stir-Fry

Preparation time: 15 minutes
Cooking time: 10 minutes
Servings: 4
Ingredients:

- 1 pound lean beef strips (such as sirloin or flank steak)
- 3 cups mixed vegetables (broccoli, bell peppers, snap peas)
- 2 tablespoons low-sodium soy sauce
- 1 tablespoon hoisin sauce
- 1 teaspoon sesame oil
- 2 cloves garlic, minced
- 1 teaspoon ginger, grated
- 2 tablespoons vegetable oil

Directions:

1. In a small bowl, mix together the low-sodium soy sauce, hoisin sauce, sesame oil, minced garlic, and grated ginger to create the sauce.
2. Heat the vegetable oil in a large skillet or wok over medium-high heat.
3. Add the beef strips to the skillet or wok and stir-fry until they are browned, removing any excess liquid if necessary.
4. Add the mixed vegetables to the skillet or wok, and continue stir-frying for 3-4 minutes until they are tender-crisp.
5. Pour the sauce over the beef and vegetables in the skillet or wok, tossing everything together to coat evenly.
6. Continue to cook for an additional 2-3 minutes until the sauce has thickened.
7. Serve the stir-fry hot, ideally with a side of brown rice or quinoa for a complete meal.

Per serving: Calories: 280kcal; Saturated fat: 2g; Sugar: 6g; Sodium: 420mg

76. Balsamic Glazed Chicken Breast

Preparation time: 10 minutes
Cooking time: 20 minutes
Servings: 4
Ingredients:

- 4 boneless, skinless chicken breasts
- 1/4 cup balsamic vinegar
- 2 tablespoons olive oil
- 2 tablespoons honey
- 2 cloves garlic, minced

- 1 teaspoon dried rosemary
- Salt and pepper to taste
- Fresh parsley for garnish (optional)

Directions:
1. In a bowl, whisk together the balsamic vinegar, olive oil, honey, minced garlic, dried rosemary, salt, and pepper to create the marinade.
2. Place the chicken breasts in a resealable plastic bag and pour half of the balsamic marinade over them, ensuring they're well coated. Marinate in the refrigerator for at least 10 minutes.
3. Heat a skillet over medium-high heat. Remove the chicken from the bag, making sure to reserve the marinade for later use.
4. Cook the chicken for 6-8 minutes per side, or until it reaches an internal temperature of 165°F and is fully cooked.
5. During the last few minutes of cooking, pour the reserved marinade into the skillet, allowing it to simmer and reduce into a glaze that coats the chicken.
6. Garnish the chicken with fresh parsley if desired, and serve immediately.

Per serving: Calories: 280kcal; Saturated fat: 2g; Sugar: 10g; Sodium: 150mg

77. Pork Stir-Fry with Broccoli and Snap Peas

Preparation time: 15 minutes
Cooking time: 15 minutes
Servings: 4
Ingredients:

- 1 pound pork loin, thinly sliced
- 2 cups broccoli florets
- 1 cup snap peas, trimmed
- 1 red bell pepper, sliced
- 2 tablespoons low-sodium soy sauce
- 1 tablespoon oyster sauce
- 1 tablespoon hoisin sauce
- 1 teaspoon sesame oil
- 2 cloves garlic, minced
- 1 teaspoon ginger, grated
- 2 tablespoons vegetable oil

Directions:
1. In a small bowl, mix together the low-sodium soy sauce, oyster sauce, hoisin sauce, sesame oil, minced garlic, and grated ginger to create the sauce.
2. Heat the vegetable oil in a large skillet or wok over medium-high heat.
3. Add the pork slices to the skillet or wok and stir-fry until they are browned and cooked through.

4. Add the broccoli florets, snap peas, and sliced red bell pepper to the skillet or wok, and continue stir-frying for an additional 3-4 minutes until the vegetables are tender-crisp.
5. Pour the prepared sauce over the pork and vegetables in the skillet or wok, tossing everything together to coat evenly.
6. Continue to cook for an additional 2-3 minutes until the sauce has thickened.
7. Serve the stir-fry hot, ideally with a side of brown rice or noodles for a complete meal.

Per serving: Calories: 320kcal; Saturated fat: 3g; Sugar: 6g; Sodium: 420mg

78. Chicken and Mushroom Skillet

Preparation time: 10 minutes
Cooking time: 20 minutes
Servings: 4
Ingredients:

- 4 boneless, skinless chicken breasts
- 8 ounces mushrooms, sliced
- 1 onion, thinly sliced
- 2 cloves garlic, minced
- 1 cup chicken broth (low-sodium)
- 1/2 cup dry white wine (optional)
- 1 teaspoon dried thyme
- Salt and pepper to taste
- 2 tablespoons olive oil
- Fresh parsley for garnish (optional)

Directions:

1. Season the chicken breasts generously with salt and pepper on both sides.
2. Heat the olive oil in a large skillet over medium-high heat.
3. Add the chicken breasts to the skillet and sear them on both sides until browned, approximately 4-5 minutes per side.
4. Remove the chicken from the skillet and set it aside on a plate.
5. In the same skillet, add the sliced mushrooms, onion, and minced garlic. Sauté for 5-7 minutes until they are softened.
6. Pour the chicken broth, white wine (if using), and dried thyme into the skillet. Bring the mixture to a simmer.
7. Return the chicken to the skillet and let it simmer for an additional 10-12 minutes, or until the chicken is fully cooked through and reaches an internal temperature of 165°F.
8. Garnish with fresh parsley if desired, and serve the chicken and mushroom skillet hot.

Per serving: Calories: 280kcal; Saturated fat: 2g; Sugar: 2g; Sodium: 250mg

79. Teriyaki Turkey Burgers

Preparation time: 15 minutes
Cooking time: 15 minutes
Servings: 4
Ingredients:

- 1 pound ground turkey
- 1/4 cup breadcrumbs
- 2 tablespoons low-sodium soy sauce
- 1 tablespoon honey
- 1 teaspoon sesame oil
- 1 teaspoon fresh ginger, grated
- 2 cloves garlic, minced
- 4 whole grain burger buns
- Lettuce, tomato, and other preferred toppings

Directions:

1. In a large bowl, combine the ground turkey, breadcrumbs, low-sodium soy sauce, honey, sesame oil, grated fresh ginger, and minced garlic. Mix until the ingredients are well combined.
2. Divide the mixture into four equal portions and shape them into burger patties.
3. Heat a grill pan over medium-high heat.
4. Grill the turkey burgers for 6-8 minutes per side, or until they are fully cooked and the internal temperature reaches 165°F.
5. Toast the burger buns on the grill for about a minute, or until they are lightly browned.
6. Assemble the burgers by placing lettuce, tomato slices, and any other preferred toppings on the toasted buns.
7. Serve the teriyaki turkey burgers immediately and enjoy.

Per serving: Calories: 300kcal; Saturated fat: 2g; Sugar: 5g; Sodium: 350mg

80. Beef and Asparagus Stir-Fry

Preparation time: 15 minutes
Cooking time: 10 minutes
Servings: 4
Ingredients:

- 1 pound lean beef strips (such as sirloin or flank steak)
- 1 bunch asparagus, that is trimmed and cut into bite-sized pieces
- 1 red bell pepper, sliced
- 2 tablespoons low-sodium soy sauce
- 1 tablespoon oyster sauce

- 1 tablespoon hoisin sauce
- 1 teaspoon sesame oil
- 2 cloves garlic, minced
- 1 teaspoon ginger, grated
- 2 tablespoons vegetable oil

Directions:
1. In a small bowl, whisk together the low-sodium soy sauce, oyster sauce, hoisin sauce, sesame oil, minced garlic, and grated ginger to create the sauce.
2. Heat the vegetable oil in a large skillet or wok over medium-high heat.
3. Add the beef strips to the skillet or wok and stir-fry until browned, draining any excess liquid if necessary.
4. Add the asparagus and sliced red bell pepper to the skillet or wok, and continue stir-frying for another 3-4 minutes until the vegetables are tender-crisp.
5. Pour the prepared sauce over the beef and vegetables in the skillet or wok, tossing everything together to ensure even coating.
6. Continue cooking for an additional 2-3 minutes, or until the sauce has thickened.
7. Serve the beef and asparagus stir-fry hot, ideally with a side of steamed rice or noodles for a complete meal.

Per serving: Calories: 320kcal; Saturated fat: 2g; Sugar: 6g; Sodium: 420mg

Ocean's Offerings: Fresh Fish Feasts for the Soul

81. Grilled Halibut with Mango Salsa

Preparation time: 15 minutes
Cooking time: 10 minutes
Servings: 4
Ingredients:

- 4 halibut fillets
- 1 mango, diced
- 1/2 red onion, finely chopped
- 1 red bell pepper, diced
- 1/4 cup fresh cilantro, chopped
- Juice of 1 lime
- Salt and pepper to taste

Directions:

1. Preheat the grill to medium-high heat.
2. Season the halibut fillets generously with salt and pepper on both sides..
3. Grill the halibut fillets for 4-5 minutes per side, or until they are fully cooked and flake easily with a fork.
4. In a bowl, combine the diced mango, finely chopped red onion, diced red bell pepper, chopped fresh cilantro, and lime juice to prepare the mango salsa.
5. Serve the grilled halibut fillets topped with the fresh mango salsa.

Per serving: Calories: 220kcal; Saturated fat: 0.5g; Sugar: 10g; Sodium: 80mg

82. Tuna Salad Lettuce Wraps

Preparation time: 10 minutes
Cooking time: 0 minutes
Servings: 2
Ingredients:

- 1 can (5 oz) tuna, drained
- 2 tbsp light mayonnaise
- 1 celery stalk, finely chopped
- 1/4 red onion, finely chopped
- 1 tsp Dijon mustard
- Salt and pepper to taste

- 4 large lettuce leaves

Directions:
1. In a bowl, combine the drained tuna, light mayonnaise, finely chopped celery, finely chopped red onion, Dijon mustard, salt, and pepper. Mix well to combine all the ingredients thoroughly.
2. Evenly spoon the tuna salad mixture onto the center of each large lettuce leaf.
3. Carefully fold or wrap the lettuce leaves around the tuna salad, securing the contents to form the lettuce wraps. Serve immediately or chill until ready to serve.

Per serving: Calories: 180kcal; Saturated fat: 0.5g; Sugar: 1g; Sodium: 320mg

83. Baked Mahi-Mahi with Lemon Butter

Preparation time: 10 minutes
Cooking time: 15 minutes
Servings: 4
Ingredients:

- 4 mahi-mahi fillets
- 2 tbsp olive oil
- 2 cloves garlic, minced
- Juice of 1 lemon
- 2 tbsp fresh parsley, chopped
- Salt and pepper to taste

Directions:
1. Preheat the oven to 400°F.
2. Place the mahi-mahi fillets in a baking dish.
3. In a small bowl, whisk together the olive oil, minced garlic, lemon juice, chopped fresh parsley, salt, and pepper. Evenly pour the mixture over the fish fillets.
4. Bake in the preheated oven for 12-15 minutes, or until the fish flakes easily with a fork, indicating it is fully cooked.

Per serving: Calories: 240kcal; Saturated fat: 1g; Sugar: 0g; Sodium: 90mg

84. Shrimp and Spinach Salad

Preparation time: 15 minutes
Cooking time: 5 minutes
Servings: 2
Ingredients:

- 8 oz shrimp, peeled and deveined
- 4 cups fresh spinach
- 1 cup cherry tomatoes, halved

- 1/4 cup feta cheese, crumbled
- 2 tbsp olive oil
- 1 tbsp balsamic vinegar
- Salt and pepper to taste

Directions:
1. Heat a pan over medium heat and sauté the shrimp in olive oil until they are pink and cooked through, about 3-5 minutes.
2. In a large bowl, combine the fresh spinach, halved cherry tomatoes, and crumbled feta cheese.
3. Add the cooked shrimp to the salad mixture.
4. Drizzle the salad with balsamic vinegar, then season with salt and pepper to taste. Toss gently to ensure all ingredients are evenly coated.

Per serving: Calories: 320kcal; Saturated fat: 3g; Sugar: 2g; Sodium: 420mg

85. Baked Cod with Herbed Breadcrumbs

Preparation time: 10 minutes
Cooking time: 15 minutes
Servings: 4
Ingredients:

- 4 cod fillets
- 1/2 cup whole wheat breadcrumbs
- 2 tbsp fresh parsley, chopped
- 1 tsp dried oregano
- 1 tsp garlic powder
- 2 tbsp olive oil
- Salt and pepper to taste
- Lemon wedges for serving

Directions:
1. Preheat the oven to 400°F.
2. Place the cod fillets on a lightly greased baking sheet.
3. In a bowl, combine the whole wheat breadcrumbs, chopped fresh parsley, dried oregano, garlic powder, olive oil, salt, and pepper.
4. Evenly press the herbed breadcrumb mixture onto the top of each cod fillet to form a crust.
5. Bake in the preheated oven for 12-15 minutes, or until the fish is opaque and flakes easily with a fork.
6. Serve the baked cod immediately, accompanied by lemon wedges for squeezing over the fish.

Per serving: Calories: 220kcal; Saturated fat: 1g; Sugar: 1g; Sodium: 180mg

86. Salmon and Asparagus Foil Packets

Preparation time: 10 minutes

Cooking time: 20 minutes

Servings: 2

Ingredients:

- 2 salmon fillets
- 1 bunch asparagus, trimmed
- 1 lemon, thinly sliced
- 2 tbsp olive oil
- 1 tsp dried dill
- Salt and pepper to taste

Directions:

1. Preheat the oven to 400°F.
2. Place each salmon fillet on a large piece of aluminum foil.
3. Arrange the trimmed asparagus around each fillet and top with thinly sliced lemon.
4. Drizzle each fillet with olive oil and evenly sprinkle with dried dill, salt, and pepper.
5. Seal the foil packets tightly to lock in moisture and flavors, then place them on a baking sheet.
6. Bake in the preheated oven for 18-20 minutes, or until the salmon is opaque and flakes easily with a fork.

Per serving: Calories: 350kcal; Saturated fat: 2g; Sugar: 2g; Sodium: 150mg

87. Tuna and White Bean Salad with Lemon Dressing

Preparation time: 15 minutes

Cooking time: 0 minutes

Servings: 4

Ingredients:

- 2 cans (5 oz each) tuna, drained
- 2 cups canned white beans, that is drained and rinsed
- 1 cucumber, diced
- 1 cup cherry tomatoes, halved
- 2 tbsp fresh parsley, chopped
- Zest and juice of 1 lemon
- 2 tbsp olive oil
- Salt and pepper to taste

Directions:

1. In a large bowl, combine the drained tuna, drained and rinsed white beans, diced cucumber, halved cherry tomatoes, and chopped fresh parsley.
2. In a small bowl, whisk together the zest and juice of one lemon, olive oil, salt, and pepper to create the dressing.
3. Drizzle the lemon dressing over the salad and toss gently to ensure all ingredients are evenly coated.

Per serving: Calories: 320kcal; Saturated fat: 1g; Sugar: 2g; Sodium: 320mg

88. Lemon Garlic Tilapia

Preparation time: 10 minutes
Cooking time: 10 minutes
Servings: 4
Ingredients:

- 4 tilapia fillets
- 2 tbsp olive oil
- 2 cloves garlic, minced
- Zest and juice of 1 lemon
- 1 tsp dried thyme
- Salt and pepper to taste
- Fresh parsley for garnish

Directions:

1. Generously season the tilapia fillets on both sides with salt, pepper, and dried thyme.
2. Heat the olive oil in a pan over medium heat. Add the minced garlic and sauté for 1-2 minutes, until fragrant but not browned.
3. Add the tilapia fillets to the pan and cook for 3-4 minutes on each side, or until the fish is opaque and flakes easily with a fork.
4. Rizzle the cooked fillets with lemon juice evenly, then sprinkle with the grated lemon zest for added flavor.
5. Garnish the fillets with chopped fresh parsley before serving for a fresh, herbal touch.

Per serving: Calories: 180kcal; Saturated fat: 1g; Sugar: 0g; Sodium: 80mg

89. Seared Scallops with Spinach and Tomato

Preparation time: 10 minutes
Cooking time: 5 minutes
Servings: 2
Ingredients:

- 10 large sea scallops
- 2 cups fresh spinach

- 1 cup cherry tomatoes, halved
- 2 tbsp olive oil
- 1 clove garlic, minced
- Salt and pepper to taste
- Lemon wedges for serving

Directions:
1. Pat the scallops dry with paper towels and season both sides with salt and pepper.
2. Heat the olive oil in a pan over medium-high heat.
3. Add the scallops to the pan and sear for 1-2 minutes on each side, or until they have a golden-brown crust.
4. Using the same pan, add the minced garlic and sauté briefly until fragrant, about 30 seconds.
5. Arrange the seared scallops over the bed of sautéed spinach and tomatoes on serving plates.
6. Serve scallops over the bed of spinach and tomatoes.
7. Squeeze fresh lemon juice over the scallops and vegetables just before serving.

Per serving: Calories: 250kcal; Saturated fat: 1g; Sugar: 2g; Sodium: 300mg

90. Baked Snapper with Citrus Glaze

Preparation time: 15 minutes
Cooking time: 20 minutes
Servings: 4
Ingredients:

- 4 snapper fillets
- 2 tbsp olive oil
- Zest and juice of 1 orange
- Zest and juice of 1 lemon
- 2 tbsp honey
- 1 tsp dried thyme
- Salt and pepper to taste
- Fresh parsley for garnish

Directions:
1. Preheat the oven to 375°F.
2. Arrange the snapper fillets in a lightly greased baking dish.
3. In a bowl, whisk together the olive oil, orange zest, orange juice, lemon zest, lemon juice, honey, dried thyme, salt, and pepper to create the citrus glaze.
4. Evenly pour or brush the citrus glaze over the snapper fillets, ensuring they are well coated.
5. Bake in the preheated oven for 18-20 minutes, or until the snapper fillets are opaque and flake easily with a fork.
6. Garnish the baked snapper with chopped fresh parsley before serving for a fresh, herbal accent.

Per serving: Calories: 280kcal; Saturated fat: 1g; Sugar: 10g; Sodium: 160mg

91. Canned Mackerel Salad

Preparation time: 10 minutes

Cooking time: 0 minutes

Servings: 2

Ingredients:

- 2 cans (5 oz each) mackerel, drained
- 1 cup cucumber, diced
- 1/2 red onion, finely chopped
- 1/4 cup black olives, sliced
- 2 tbsp olive oil
- Zest and juice of 1 lemon
- Salt and pepper to taste

Directions:

1. In a large bowl, combine the drained mackerel, diced cucumber, finely chopped red onion, and sliced black olives.
2. In a small bowl, whisk together the olive oil, zest and juice of one lemon, salt, and pepper to create the dressing.
3. Drizzle the dressing over the mackerel salad and toss gently to ensure all the ingredients are evenly coated.

Per serving: Calories: 320kcal; Saturated fat: 1g; Sugar: 2g; Sodium: 480mg

92. Grilled Sardines with Herbs

Preparation time: 15 minutes

Cooking time: 8 minutes

Servings: 4

Ingredients:

- 8 fresh sardines, cleaned and gutted
- 2 tbsp olive oil
- 2 cloves garlic, minced
- 1 tbsp fresh rosemary, chopped
- 1 tbsp fresh thyme, chopped
- Salt and pepper to taste
- Lemon wedges for serving

Directions:
1. Preheat the grill to medium-high heat.
2. Gently rub the sardines with olive oil, then season them evenly with minced garlic, chopped fresh rosemary, chopped fresh thyme, salt, and pepper.
3. Place the sardines on the grill and cook for 3-4 minutes on each side, or until they are thoroughly cooked and the skin is slightly charred.
4. Serve the grilled sardines immediately, accompanied by fresh lemon wedges for squeezing over the fish.

Per serving: Calories: 220kcal; Saturated fat: 1g; Sugar: 0g; Sodium: 300mg

93. Tuna and Cucumber Roll-Ups

Preparation time: 10 minutes

Cooking time: 0 minutes

Servings: 2

Ingredients:

- 1 can (5 oz) tuna, drained
- 1/4 cup Greek yogurt
- 1 tbsp Dijon mustard
- 1 cucumber, thinly sliced lengthwise
- 1 carrot, julienned
- Fresh parsley for garnish
- Salt and pepper to taste

Directions:
1. In a bowl, combine the drained tuna, Greek yogurt, Dijon mustard, salt, and pepper. Mix well to create a creamy tuna filling.
2. Lay the thinly sliced cucumber strips flat on a work surface and place a spoonful of the tuna mixture near one end of each slice.
3. Place a few strands of julienned carrot on top of the tuna mixture on each cucumber slice.
4. Carefully roll up the cucumber slices, starting from the end with the tuna, and secure each roll with a toothpick to hold it together.
5. Garnish each tuna and cucumber roll-up with a small sprig of fresh parsley before serving.

Per serving: Calories: 180kcal; Saturated fat: 0.5g; Sugar: 3g; Sodium: 320mg

94. Lemon Dill Mackerel

Preparation time: 10 minutes
Cooking time: 5 minutes
Servings: 2
Ingredients:

- 2 mackerel fillets
- 2 tbsp olive oil
- Zest and juice of 1 lemon
- 1 tbsp fresh dill, chopped
- 1 clove garlic, minced
- Salt and pepper to taste

Directions:

1. Generously season the mackerel fillets on both sides with salt and pepper.
2. In a small bowl, whisk together the olive oil, lemon zest, lemon juice, chopped fresh dill, and minced garlic to create the lemon dill sauce.
3. Heat a pan over medium-high heat, then place the mackerel fillets in the pan, cooking for 2-3 minutes on each side, or until golden brown and cooked through.
4. Just before serving, drizzle the prepared lemon dill sauce evenly over the cooked mackerel fillets.

Per serving: Calories: 280kcal; Saturated fat: 2g; Sugar: 0g; Sodium: 120mg

95. Swordfish and Vegetable Kebabs

Preparation time: 15 minutes
Cooking time: 10 minutes
Servings: 4
Ingredients:

- 1 lb swordfish, cut into cubes
- 1 bell pepper, cut into chunks
- 1 zucchini, sliced
- 1 red onion, cut into wedges
- 2 tbsp olive oil
- 1 tsp dried oregano
- 1 tsp paprika
- Salt and pepper to taste

Directions:

1. Preheat the grill to medium-high heat.
2. Alternately thread the swordfish cubes, bell pepper chunks, zucchini slices, and red onion wedges onto skewers.

3. In a small bowl, whisk together the olive oil, dried oregano, paprika, salt, and pepper to create a marinade.
4. Generously brush the kebabs on all sides with the olive oil mixture, ensuring they are well coated.
5. Grill the kebabs for 8-10 minutes, turning occasionally, until the swordfish is cooked through and the vegetables are tender and slightly charred.

Per serving: Calories: 320kcal; Saturated fat: 1g; Sugar: 3g; Sodium: 200mg

96. Baked Trout with Almond Crust

Preparation time: 15 minutes

Cooking time: 15 minutes

Servings: 2

Ingredients:

- 2 trout fillets
- 1/4 cup almonds, finely chopped
- 1 tbsp whole wheat flour
- 1 tbsp Dijon mustard
- 1 tbsp olive oil
- 1 tsp lemon zest
- Salt and pepper to taste

Directions:

1. Preheat the oven to 400°F.
2. In a medium bowl, combine the finely chopped almonds, whole wheat flour, Dijon mustard, olive oil, lemon zest, salt, and pepper, mixing well to create the crust mixture.
3. Arrange the trout fillets on a lightly greased baking sheet. Evenly press the almond mixture onto the top surface of each fillet to form a crust.
4. Bake in the preheated oven for 12-15 minutes, or until the trout is cooked through and the almond crust is golden and crispy.

Per serving: Calories: 280kcal; Saturated fat: 1g; Sugar: 0g; Sodium: 120mg

97. Seared Tuna with Sesame Seeds

Preparation time: 10 minutes

Cooking time: 3 minutes

Servings: 2

Ingredients:

- 2 tuna steaks
- 2 tbsp soy sauce (low-sodium)
- 1 tbsp sesame oil
- 2 tbsp sesame seeds

- 1 tbsp olive oil
- 1 green onion, finely chopped (for garnish)

Directions:
1. Pat the tuna steaks dry with paper towels, then lightly brush them on all sides with low-sodium soy sauce.
2. Press the tuna steaks into the sesame seeds, ensuring they are evenly coated on all sides.
3. Heat the olive oil in a pan over high heat until hot but not smoking.
4. Sear the tuna steaks for 1.5 minutes on each side, achieving a rare center while ensuring a golden crust.
5. After searing, lightly drizzle sesame oil over the tuna steaks to enhance their flavor.
6. Garnish the seared tuna steaks with finely chopped green onions before serving for a fresh touch.

Per serving: Calories: 220kcal; Saturated fat: 1g; Sugar: 0g; Sodium: 320mg

98. Lemon Buttered Catfish

Preparation time: 10 minutes
Cooking time: 10 minutes
Servings: 2
Ingredients:

- 2 catfish fillets
- 2 tbsp butter
- Juice of 1 lemon
- 1 tsp dried thyme
- 1 clove garlic, minced
- Salt and pepper to taste
- Fresh parsley for garnish

Directions:
1. Generously season both sides of the catfish fillets with salt, pepper, and dried thyme.
2. Melt the butter in a pan over medium heat until it starts to bubble lightly.
3. Add the minced garlic to the melted butter and sauté for 1-2 minutes, until fragrant but not browned.
4. Carefully add the catfish fillets to the pan and cook for 4-5 minutes on each side, or until the fish flakes easily with a fork and is opaque throughout.
5. Drizzle lemon juice over the catfish and garnish with fresh parsley before serving.

Per serving: Calories: 280kcal; Saturated fat: 3g; Sugar: 0g; Sodium: 240mg

99. Sardine and Olive Tapenade

Preparation time: 10 minutes

Cooking time: 0 minutes

Servings: 4

Ingredients:

- 1 can (4 oz) sardines in olive oil, drained
- 1/2 cup Kalamata olives, pitted
- 2 tbsp capers
- 1 clove garlic, minced
- 1 tbsp fresh parsley, chopped
- 2 tbsp olive oil
- Juice of 1 lemon
- Salt and pepper to taste
- Whole grain crackers or sliced cucumber for serving

Directions:

1. In a food processor, combine the drained sardines, pitted Kalamata olives, capers, minced garlic, and chopped fresh parsley.
2. Pulse the mixture until it reaches a finely chopped consistency, suitable for spreading.
3. Transfer the tapenade mixture to a bowl, then gently stir in the olive oil, fresh lemon juice, and season with salt and pepper to taste.
4. Serve the tapenade accompanied by whole grain crackers or freshly sliced cucumber for dipping.

Per serving: Calories: 180kcal; Saturated fat: 2g; Sugar: 0g; Sodium: 480mg

100. Baked Haddock with Lemon Pepper

Preparation time: 10 minutes

Cooking time: 15 minutes

Servings: 2

Ingredients:

- 2 haddock fillets
- 2 tbsp olive oil
- Zest and juice of 1 lemon
- 1 tsp black pepper
- 1 tsp dried thyme
- 1/2 tsp garlic powder
- Salt to taste
- Fresh dill for garnish

Directions:
1. Preheat the oven to 400°F.
2. Arrange the haddock fillets in a lightly greased baking dish.
3. In a small bowl, whisk together the olive oil, lemon zest, lemon juice, black pepper, dried thyme, garlic powder, and salt to create the seasoning mixture.
4. Evenly spoon or brush the lemon pepper mixture over the haddock fillets, ensuring they are well coated.
5. Bake in the preheated oven for 12-15 minutes, or until the haddock flakes easily with a fork and is opaque throughout.
6. Garnish the baked haddock with fresh dill sprigs before serving for an added touch of freshness.

Per serving: Calories: 280kcal; Saturated fat: 2g; Sugar: 0g; Sodium: 220mg

Perfect Pairings: Sides & Sauces to Elevate Every Dish

101. Roasted Cauliflower with Turmeric

Preparation time: 10 minutes

Cooking time: 25 minutes

Servings: 4

Ingredients:

- 1 head cauliflower, cut into florets
- 2 tablespoons olive oil
- 1 teaspoon turmeric
- 1 teaspoon cumin
- Salt and pepper to taste
- Fresh parsley for garnish (optional)

Directions:

1. Preheat the oven to 425°F.
2. In a large bowl, toss the cauliflower florets with olive oil, turmeric, cumin, salt, and pepper until they are evenly coated.
3. Spread the cauliflower florets on a baking sheet in a single layer to ensure even roasting.
4. Roast in the preheated oven for 20-25 minutes, or until the cauliflower is golden brown and tender, turning the florets halfway through the cooking time.
5. Garnish the roasted cauliflower with fresh parsley for a burst of color and flavor before serving, if desired.

Per serving: Calories: 80kcal; Saturated fat: 1g; Sugar: 3g; Sodium: 30mg

102. Green Beans with Toasted Almonds and Lemon Zest

Preparation time: 10 minutes

Cooking time: 10 minutes

Servings: 4

Ingredients:

- 1 lb green beans, trimmed
- 2 tablespoons olive oil
- 1/4 cup sliced almonds
- 1 teaspoon lemon zest
- 2 tablespoons lemon juice
- Salt and pepper to taste
- 2 cloves garlic, minced

Directions:

1. Bring a large pot of salted water to a boil. Add the green beans and cook until they are bright green and tender, about 5 minutes. Drain well and set aside.
2. In a large skillet, heat the olive oil over medium heat. Add the sliced almonds and toast them, stirring frequently, until golden and fragrant, about 3 minutes.
3. Add the minced garlic to the skillet and sauté for about 30 seconds, or until fragrant.
4. Add the cooked green beans, lemon zest, and lemon juice to the skillet. Toss to combine and heat through. Season with salt and pepper to taste.
5. Transfer the green beans to a serving dish. Serve warm or at room temperature.

Per serving: Calories: 120kcal; Saturated fat: 1g; Sugar: 4g; Sodium: 30mg

103. Sautéed Swiss Chard with Garlic

Preparation time: 10 minutes
Cooking time: 8 minutes
Servings: 4
Ingredients:

- 1 bunch Swiss chard, washed and chopped
- 1 tablespoon olive oil
- 2 cloves garlic, minced
- Crushed red pepper flakes (optional)
- Salt and pepper to taste
- Lemon wedges for garnish (optional)

Directions:

1. Heat the olive oil in a large skillet over medium heat. Add the minced garlic and sauté for 1-2 minutes, or until it becomes fragrant.
2. Add the chopped Swiss chard to the skillet. Cook it, stirring occasionally, for about 5-7 minutes, or until it has wilted but retains a vibrant green color.
3. Season the chard with salt, pepper, and optional red pepper flakes to taste.
4. Transfer the sautéed chard to a serving dish. If desired, garnish with lemon wedges before serving.

Per serving: Calories: 60kcal; Saturated fat: 1g; Sugar: 1g; Sodium: 35mg

104. Brown Rice and Black Beans

Preparation time: 10 minutes
Cooking time: 45 minutes
Servings: 4
Ingredients:

- 1 cup brown rice, rinsed
- 2 cups water

- 1 can (15 oz) black beans, that is drained and rinsed
- 1 teaspoon cumin
- 1 teaspoon chili powder
- Salt and pepper to taste
- Fresh cilantro for garnish (optional)

Directions:
1. Combine the brown rice and water in a saucepan. Bring to a boil, then reduce the heat to low, cover, and simmer for 40-45 minutes, or until the rice is tender and the water has been absorbed.
2. In a separate pot, combine the black beans, cumin, chili powder, salt, and pepper. Cook over medium heat until heated through.
3. Combine the cooked black beans with the cooked brown rice, mixing well.
4. Garnish with fresh cilantro if desired, and serve.

Per serving: Calories: 250kcal; Saturated fat: 0.5g; Sugar: 1g; Sodium: 10mg

105. Roasted Eggplant with Tahini Sauce

Preparation time: 15 minutes
Cooking time: 25 minutes
Servings: 4
Ingredients:

- 1 large eggplant, sliced into 1/2-inch rounds
- 2 tablespoons olive oil
- Salt and pepper to taste
- 1/4 cup tahini
- 2 tablespoons lemon juice
- 1 clove garlic, minced
- Fresh parsley for garnish (optional)

Directions:
1. Preheat the oven to 400°F.
2. Arrange the eggplant slices on a baking sheet. Brush both sides of each slice with olive oil, and then season with salt and pepper.
3. Roast in the preheated oven for 20-25 minutes, turning the slices over halfway through the cooking time, until they are golden brown and tender.
4. In a bowl, whisk together the tahini, lemon juice, and minced garlic until well combined.
5. Evenly drizzle the tahini sauce over the roasted eggplant. If desired, garnish with fresh parsley before serving.

Per serving: Calories: 180kcal; Saturated fat: 1g; Sugar: 3g; Sodium: 15mg

106. Mashed Butternut Squash

Preparation time: 15 minutes
Cooking time: 25 minutes
Servings: 4
Ingredients:

- 1 medium butternut squash, that is peeled, seeded, and diced
- 1 tablespoon olive oil
- Salt and pepper to taste
- 2 tablespoons unsalted butter
- 1/4 cup low-fat milk

Directions:

1. Steam or boil the diced butternut squash until fork-tender, about 20-25 minutes.
2. After draining the squash, use a potato masher or fork to thoroughly mash it.
3. Heat the olive oil in a pan over medium heat. Then add the mashed butternut squash, seasoning with salt and pepper as you stir everything together.
4. Incorporate the butter and milk into the squash, mashing and stirring until the mixture is smooth and evenly combined.
5. Taste and adjust the seasoning with additional salt and pepper if needed before serving.

Per serving: Calories: 120kcal; Saturated fat: 3g; Sugar: 3g; Sodium: 15mg

107. Sautéed Spinach with Pine Nuts

Preparation time: 10 minutes
Cooking time: 5 minutes
Servings: 4
Ingredients:

- 1 tablespoon olive oil
- 1 pound fresh spinach, washed and stems removed
- 2 tablespoons pine nuts
- 1 clove garlic, minced
- Salt and pepper to taste
- Lemon wedges for garnish (optional)

Directions:

1. Warm the olive oil in a large skillet on medium heat before adding the pine nuts. Toast the nuts until they achieve a light golden color, which should take approximately 1 to 2 minutes.
2. Add the minced garlic to the skillet and sauté for 1 minute, or until it becomes fragrant.
3. Incorporate the fresh spinach into the skillet, tossing it gently until it wilts.
4. Season the spinach with salt and pepper, adjusting to taste.

5. Transfer the sautéed spinach to a serving dish. If desired, garnish with lemon wedges before serving.

Per serving: Calories: 80kcal; Saturated fat: 1g; Sugar: 1g; Sodium: 50mg

108. Steamed Artichokes with Lemon Butter

Preparation time: 15 minutes
Cooking time: 45 minutes
Servings: 4
Ingredients:

- 4 large artichokes
- 1 lemon, sliced
- 1/4 cup unsalted butter, melted
- Salt and pepper to taste

Directions:

1. Trim the stem of each artichoke and remove the tough outer leaves.
2. Remove the top third of each artichoke and trim the sharp tips from the remaining leaves using kitchen scissors for safety and ease.
3. Set a steamer basket inside a large pot filled with water, add lemon slices, and bring it to a simmer.
4. Place the artichokes in the steamer basket, cover the pot, and steam for 40-45 minutes, or until the leaves pull away easily.
5. In a small bowl, combine the melted butter with a squeeze of fresh lemon juice, and season with salt and pepper to taste.
6. Serve the artichokes warm, accompanied by the lemon butter sauce for dipping.

Per serving: Calories: 160kcal; Saturated fat: 8g; Sugar: 2g; Sodium: 40mg

109. Cilantro Lime Brown Rice

Preparation time: 5 minutes
Cooking time: 40 minutes
Servings: 4
Ingredients:

- 1 cup brown rice
- 2 cups water
- 1 tablespoon olive oil
- Zest and juice of 1 lime
- 2 tablespoons fresh cilantro, chopped
- Salt to taste

Directions:

1. Combine the brown rice and water in a saucepan. Bring to a boil, then lower the heat to a simmer, cover, and cook for 35-40 minutes, or until the rice is tender and the water has been fully absorbed.
2. Once cooked, fluff the rice with a fork to separate the grains for a lighter texture.
3. In a separate bowl, combine the olive oil, lime zest, lime juice, and chopped cilantro, mixing well.
4. Drizzle the cilantro lime mixture over the cooked rice, tossing thoroughly to ensure the rice is evenly coated with the flavors.
5. Season the rice with salt according to your preference, then serve immediately.

Per serving: Calories: 180kcal; Saturated fat: 1g; Sugar: 0g; Sodium: 5mg

110. Roasted Brussels Sprouts with Balsamic Glaze

Preparation time: 10 minutes

Cooking time: 25 minutes

Servings: 4

Ingredients:

- 1 pound Brussels sprouts, trimmed and halved
- 2 tablespoons olive oil
- Salt and pepper to taste
- 2 tablespoons balsamic glaze

Directions:

1. Preheat the oven to 400°F.
2. On a baking sheet, evenly coat the Brussels sprouts with olive oil, and season with salt and pepper to taste.
3. Roast in the preheated oven for 20-25 minutes, or until the Brussels sprouts are golden brown and crispy at the edges.
4. Before serving, evenly drizzle the balsamic glaze over the roasted Brussels sprouts for a rich, caramelized finish.

Per serving: Calories: 120kcal; Saturated fat: 2g; Sugar: 6g; Sodium: 30mg

Sweet Temptations: Guiltless Treats for Dessert Lovers

111. Baked Pear with Cinnamon and Almonds

Preparation time: 10 minutes

Cooking time: 20 minutes

Servings: 2

Ingredients:

- 2 ripe pears, halved and cored
- 1 teaspoon cinnamon
- 2 tablespoons chopped almonds
- 1 tablespoon honey (optional)

Directions:

1. Preheat the oven to 375°F.
2. Arrange the pear halves cut-side up on a baking sheet..
3. Evenly sprinkle the cinnamon over the pear halves and then distribute the chopped almonds atop each one.
4. Bake in the preheated oven for 20 minutes, or until the pears become tender and slightly golden.
5. If using, lightly drizzle honey over the baked pears just before serving for added sweetness.

Per serving: Calories: 150kcal; Saturated fat: 0.5g; Sugar: 12g; Sodium: 0mg

112. Banana and Walnut Muffins

Preparation time: 15 minutes

Cooking time: 20 minutes

Servings: 12

Ingredients:

- 2 ripe bananas, mashed
- 1/4 cup melted coconut oil
- 1/4 cup honey
- 2 large eggs
- 1 teaspoon vanilla extract
- 1 3/4 cups whole wheat flour
- 1 teaspoon baking soda
- 1/2 teaspoon salt
- 1/2 cup chopped walnuts

Directions:

1. Preheat the oven to 350°F and prepare a muffin tin by lining it with paper liners.
2. In a large bowl, combine the mashed bananas, melted coconut oil, honey, eggs, and vanilla extract until well mixed.
3. In another bowl, whisk the whole wheat flour, baking soda, and salt together.
4. Gently mix the wet and dry ingredients until just combined, then carefully fold in the chopped walnuts.
5. Evenly distribute the batter among the muffin cups, then bake for 20 minutes, or until a toothpick inserted into the center of a muffin comes out clean.

Per serving: Calories: 150kcal; Saturated fat: 1g; Sugar: 8g; Sodium: 150mg

113. Chocolate Avocado Mousse

Preparation time: 10 minutes
Cooking time: 0 minutes
Servings: 4
Ingredients:

- 2 ripe avocados
- 1/4 cup cocoa powder
- 1/4 cup honey or maple syrup
- 1 teaspoon vanilla extract
- Pinch of salt
- 1/4 cup almond milk

Directions:

1. In a blender or food processor, combine the avocados, cocoa powder, honey (or maple syrup), vanilla extract, salt, and almond milk.
2. Blend until the mixture is completely smooth and creamy.
3. Evenly divide the mousse into serving cups and refrigerate for at least 2 hours to allow it to set before serving.

Per serving: Calories: 200kcal; Saturated fat: 2g; Sugar: 10g; Sodium: 5mg

114. Apple Cinnamon Baked Oatmeal

Preparation time: 10 minutes
Cooking time: 30 minutes
Servings: 4
Ingredients:

- 2 cups old-fashioned oats
- 1 teaspoon baking powder
- 1/2 teaspoon cinnamon

- 1/4 teaspoon salt
- 1.5 cups unsweetened almond milk
- 1/4 cup honey or maple syrup
- 1 large egg, beaten
- 1 teaspoon vanilla extract
- 2 medium apples, peeled, cored, and diced
- Chopped nuts for topping (optional)

Directions:
1. Preheat the oven to 350°F and lightly grease a baking dish with cooking spray or a dab of oil.
2. In a large bowl, combine the oats, baking powder, cinnamon, and salt.
3. In a separate bowl, whisk the almond milk, honey (or maple syrup), beaten egg, and vanilla extract together.
4. Gently mix the wet ingredients into the dry ingredients until just combined, then carefully fold in the diced apples.
5. Pour the oatmeal mixture into the prepared baking dish and bake for 30 minutes, or until the top is golden brown and the oatmeal is set.
6. Let the baked oatmeal cool for a few minutes before serving. If desired, sprinkle with chopped nuts for added crunch.

Per serving: Calories: 250kcal; Saturated fat: 1g; Sugar: 10g; Sodium: 150mg

115. Berry and Yogurt Parfait

Preparation time: 5 minutes
Cooking time: 0 minutes
Servings: 2
Ingredients:

- 1 cup mixed berries (strawberries, blueberries, raspberries)
- 1 cup low-fat Greek yogurt
- 1/4 cup granola (look for low-sugar options)

Directions:
1. In serving glasses or bowls, begin by layering a spoonful of Greek yogurt, followed by a layer of mixed berries.
2. Continue layering the yogurt and berries, ending with a generous sprinkle of granola on the top for a crunchy finish.
3. Serve the parfait immediately to enjoy its refreshing taste and satisfying texture.

Per serving: Calories: 200kcal; Saturated fat: 0.5g; Sugar: 8g; Sodium: 50mg

116. Baked Peaches with Almond Crumble

Preparation time: 10 minutes
Cooking time: 20 minutes
Servings: 4
Ingredients:

- 4 ripe peaches, halved and pitted
- 1/4 cup almond flour
- 2 tablespoons rolled oats
- 2 tablespoons chopped almonds
- 1 tablespoon honey
- 1/2 teaspoon cinnamon

Directions:

1. Preheat the oven to 375°F.
2. Arrange the peach halves cut-side up in a baking dish.
3. In a medium bowl, combine the almond flour, rolled oats, chopped almonds, honey, and cinnamon until well mixed.
4. Evenly distribute the crumble mixture over each peach half, gently pressing to adhere.
5. Bake for 20 minutes, or until the peaches have softened and the crumble topping is golden brown.

Per serving: Calories: 150kcal; Saturated fat: 0.5g; Sugar: 12g; Sodium: 0mg

117. Strawberry and Banana Popsicles

Preparation time: 10 minutes
Cooking time: 0 minutes
Servings: 6
Ingredients:

- 1 cup strawberries, hulled
- 2 ripe bananas
- 1 cup unsweetened almond milk
- 1 teaspoon vanilla extract

Directions:

1. Combine the strawberries, ripe bananas, unsweetened almond milk, and vanilla extract in a blender. Blend until the mixture is completely smooth.
2. Pour the blended mixture evenly into the popsicle molds.
3. Carefully insert popsicle sticks into the center of each mold. Freeze the molds for at least 4 hours, or until the popsicles are fully set and firm.
4. To release the popsicles, run the outside of the molds under warm water for a few seconds until they can be easily removed.

Per serving: Calories: 50kcal; Saturated fat: 0g; Sugar: 6g; Sodium: 0mg

118. Lemon Poppy Seed Muffins

Preparation time: 15 minutes
Cooking time: 20 minutes
Servings: 12
Ingredients:

- 2 cups almond flour
- 1/4 cup coconut flour
- 1/2 teaspoon baking soda
- 1/4 teaspoon salt
- Zest and juice of 2 lemons
- 1/4 cup melted coconut oil
- 1/4 cup honey or maple syrup
- 3 large eggs
- 1 teaspoon vanilla extract
- 1 tablespoon poppy seeds

Directions:

1. Preheat the oven to 350°F then line a muffin tin using paper liners.
2. In a large mixing bowl, thoroughly whisk together the almond flour, coconut flour, baking soda, and salt to ensure an even distribution of ingredients.
3. In a separate bowl, combine the lemon zest, lemon juice, melted coconut oil, honey (or maple syrup), eggs, and vanilla extract, mixing well to create a homogeneous wet mixture.
4. Gradually mix the wet ingredients into the dry ingredients until just combined, then gently fold in the poppy seeds to avoid overmixing.
5. Evenly distribute the batter among the lined muffin cups, filling each about three-quarters full. Bake for 20 minutes or until a toothpick inserted into the center of a muffin comes out clean.

Per serving: Calories: 180kcal; Saturated fat: 2g; Sugar: 5g; Sodium: 100mg

119. Chocolate Covered Almonds

Preparation time: 10 minutes
Cooking time: 5 minutes
Servings: 4
Ingredients:

- 1 cup raw almonds
- 1/2 cup dark chocolate chips (above 70% cocoa)
- 1 teaspoon coconut oil
- Sea salt for sprinkling (optional)

Directions:

1. Gently melt the dark chocolate chips with the coconut oil in a double boiler or microwave, stirring frequently until the mixture is smooth and glossy.
2. Fold the raw almonds into the melted chocolate, ensuring each almond is thoroughly coated for an even layer of chocolate.
3. With a spoon, carefully drop clusters of the chocolate-covered almonds onto a tray lined with parchment paper, allowing for individual treats.
4. Lightly sprinkle sea salt over the chocolate-covered almonds, if using, then allow them to cool at room temperature or in the refrigerator until the chocolate sets firmly.

Per serving: Calories: 200kcal; Saturated fat: 3g; Sugar: 5g; Sodium: 5mg

120. Greek Yogurt and Berry Bark

Preparation time: 10 minutes
Cooking time: 0 minutes
Servings: 8
Ingredients:

- 2 cups plain Greek yogurt
- 1 tablespoon honey or maple syrup
- 1 cup mixed berries (strawberries, blueberries, raspberries)

Directions:

1. In a medium-sized bowl, thoroughly combine the Greek yogurt with honey or maple syrup until smooth.
2. Line a baking sheet with parchment paper, then evenly spread the yogurt mixture across the surface, creating a smooth layer.
3. Evenly distribute the mixed berries on top of the yogurt layer, ensuring a colorful and balanced distribution.
4. Freeze the tray for a minimum of 3 hours to solidify. Once set, break the yogurt bark into pieces of varying sizes for serving.

Per serving: Calories: 100kcal; Saturated fat: 1g; Sugar: 4g; Sodium: 20mg

121. Coconut and Chia Seed Pudding

Preparation time: 5 minutes
Cooking time: 0 minutes
Servings: 4
Ingredients:

- 1 can (14 oz) light coconut milk
- 1/4 cup chia seeds
- 1 tablespoon honey or maple syrup

- 1/2 teaspoon vanilla extract
- Unsweetened shredded coconut for topping (optional)

Directions:
1. In a large mixing bowl, thoroughly combine the coconut milk, chia seeds, honey (or maple syrup), and vanilla extract using a whisk.
2. Cover the bowl with a lid or plastic wrap and refrigerate to allow the pudding to thicken, ideally overnight. Stir the mixture once or twice during this period to ensure even thickening.
3. Give the pudding a final stir to ensure a smooth consistency. Serve in individual bowls, garnished with a sprinkle of unsweetened shredded coconut, if preferred.

Per serving: Calories: 150kcal; Saturated fat: 4g; Sugar: 3g; Sodium: 10mg

122. Baked Apple Chips

Preparation time: 10 minutes
Cooking time: 2 hours
Servings: 4
Ingredients:

- 2 large apples, thinly sliced
- Cinnamon for sprinkling (optional)

Directions:
1. Preheat your oven to 200°F. Prepare a baking sheet by lining it with parchment paper to prevent sticking.
2. Lay out the apple slices on the prepared baking sheet, ensuring they are in a single layer to promote even baking.
3. For those who enjoy a hint of spice, lightly dust the apple slices with cinnamon before baking.
4. Bake the apple slices for 2 hours, or until they are completely crisp. Remember to flip each slice halfway through the baking time to ensure they crisp up evenly.
5. Allow the apple chips to cool on the baking sheet for a few minutes after baking. This will help them to crisp up further before serving.

Per serving: Calories: 50kcal; Saturated fat: 0g; Sugar: 10g; Sodium: 0mg

123. Pineapple and Coconut Frozen Yogurt

Preparation time: 10 minutes
Cooking time: 0 minutes
Servings: 4
Ingredients:

- 2 cups plain Greek yogurt
- 1 cup frozen pineapple chunks
- 1/4 cup shredded coconut

- 1 tablespoon honey or maple syrup

Directions:
1. In a blender, combine the Greek yogurt, frozen pineapple chunks, shredded coconut, and your choice of honey or maple syrup.
2. Blend the mixture until it reaches a smooth and creamy consistency.
3. Transfer the blended mixture into a shallow dish and freeze for a minimum of 4 hours to achieve the desired frozen yogurt texture.
4. Once frozen, scoop the yogurt into bowls or cones and garnish with extra shredded coconut for an additional tropical flair.

Per serving: Calories: 120kcal; Saturated fat: 3g; Sugar: 8g; Sodium: 30mg

124. Mixed Fruit Sorbet

Preparation time: 10 minutes
Cooking time: 0 minutes
Servings: 4
Ingredients:

- 2 cups mixed frozen fruits (berries, mango, pineapple)
- 1/4 cup water
- Juice of 1 lemon

Directions:
1. Combine the mixed frozen fruits, water, and lemon juice in a blender.
2. Pulse until you achieve a smooth and homogeneous mixture.
3. Transfer the blended fruit mixture into a shallow dish and freeze for a minimum of 4 hours to solidify.
4. Allow the sorbet to rest at room temperature for a few minutes prior to serving for easier scooping.

Per serving: Calories: 70kcal; Saturated fat: 0g; Sugar: 10g; Sodium: 0mg

125. Pumpkin and Walnut Bites

Preparation time: 15 minutes
Cooking time: 0 minutes
Servings: 12
Ingredients:

- 1 cup canned pumpkin puree
- 1/4 cup almond flour
- 1/4 cup chopped walnuts
- 2 tablespoons ground flaxseed
- 1 teaspoon cinnamon
- 1/2 teaspoon nutmeg

- 1 tablespoon honey or maple syrup

Directions:
1. Combine the pumpkin puree, almond flour, chopped walnuts, ground flaxseed, cinnamon, nutmeg, and honey or maple syrup in a large mixing bowl.
2. Chill the mixture in the refrigerator for 30 minutes to firm up, making it easier to roll into balls.
3. Form the chilled mixture into bite-sized balls and place them back in the refrigerator until you're ready to serve.

Per serving: Calories: 60kcal; Saturated fat: 0.5g; Sugar: 2g; Sodium: 5mg

Sips of Serenity: Refreshing Beverages for Every Mood

126. Herbal Infusion with Mint and Ginger

Preparation time: 5 minutes

Cooking time: 0 minutes

Servings: 1

Ingredients:

- 1 herbal tea bag (such as chamomile or peppermint)
- 1 slice of fresh ginger
- 5-6 fresh mint leaves
- 1 cup boiling water

Directions:

1. In a large mug, add the herbal tea bag along with the slice of fresh ginger and mint leaves.
2. Carefully pour freshly boiled water into the mug, ensuring all ingredients are submerged.
3. Let the tea steep for 3-5 minutes, adjusting the time based on desired strength.
4. Discard the tea bag after steeping and savor the warm, aromatic herbal infusion.

Per serving: Calories: 0kcal; Saturated fat: 0g; Sugar: 0g; Sodium: 0mg

127. Cranberry and Orange Smoothie

Preparation time: 8 minutes

Cooking time: 0 minutes

Servings: 2

Ingredients:

- 1 cup fresh or frozen cranberries
- 1 orange, peeled and segmented
- 1 banana
- 1 cup low-fat yogurt
- Ice cubes (optional)

Directions:

1. In a blender, combine the cranberries, orange segments, banana, and yogurt.
2. Blend on high speed until the mixture becomes smooth and creamy.
3. If a colder consistency is preferred, add ice cubes and blend until smooth.
4. Divide the smoothie evenly between two glasses and serve immediately for a refreshing treat.

Per serving: Calories: 120kcal; Saturated fat: 0.5g; Sugar: 15g; Sodium: 35mg

128. Cucumber and Mint Cooler

Preparation time: 5 minutes

Cooking time: 0 minutes

Servings: 1

Ingredients:

- 1/2 cucumber, thinly sliced
- 5-6 fresh mint leaves
- 1 tablespoon lime juice
- 1 cup cold water
- Ice cubes

Directions:

1. Place the cucumber slices and mint leaves in a tall glass.
2. Pour the lime juice followed by the cold water into the glass.
3. Stir the mixture vigorously to infuse the flavors, then add ice cubes to chill.
4. Serve immediately to enjoy the maximum refreshing effect of your cucumber and mint cooler.

Per serving: Calories: 10kcal; Saturated fat: 0g; Sugar: 2g; Sodium: 2mg

129. Cherry and Pomegranate Iced Tea

Preparation time: 10 minutes

Cooking time: 5 minutes (for steeping)

Servings: 2

Ingredients:

- 2 black tea bags
- 1 cup fresh or frozen cherries, pitted
- 1/2 cup pomegranate seeds
- Ice cubes

Directions:

1. Steep the black tea bags in boiling water for exactly 5 minutes to extract full flavor without bitterness.
2. After removing the tea bags, allow the tea to cool at room temperature, avoiding rapid temperature changes to preserve the tea's flavor.
3. In a large pitcher, gently mix the cooled tea with the cherries and pomegranate seeds, allowing the fruits to infuse their flavors.
4. Chill the tea mixture in the refrigerator for at least 2 hours, or until thoroughly cold, to enhance the infusion of fruit flavors.
5. Fill glasses with ice, pour the chilled Cherry and Pomegranate Iced Tea over, and enjoy immediately for a refreshing experience.

Per serving: Calories: 20kcal; Saturated fat: 0g; Sugar: 3g; Sodium: 5mg

130. Kiwi and Spinach Smoothie

Preparation time: 5 minutes

Cooking time: 0 minutes

Servings: 2

Ingredients:

- 2 kiwis, peeled and sliced
- 1 cup fresh spinach leaves
- 1 banana
- 1/2 cup plain Greek yogurt
- 1 cup water
- Ice cubes (optional)

Directions:

1. Place the kiwi slices, fresh spinach leaves, banana, Greek yogurt, and water into the blender, ensuring they are evenly distributed for a smooth blend.
2. Blend the ingredients on high speed until the mixture reaches a creamy and smooth consistency, with no visible spinach pieces.
3. If a cooler texture is preferred, add ice cubes to the blender and pulse until the ice is fully incorporated and the smoothie is chilled.
4. Divide the smoothie evenly among two glasses, garnish with a slice of kiwi if desired, and enjoy immediately for the best taste and nutritional benefits.

Per serving: Calories: 120kcal; Saturated fat: 0.5g; Sugar: 12g; Sodium: 25mg

12-Week Meal Plan with Downloadable Shopping Lists

Welcome to your journey with my *DASH Diet Cookbook for Beginners*. I've developed a meal plan to kickstart your adherence to the DASH diet, aimed at managing blood pressure and fostering a heart-healthy lifestyle.

This cookbook is designed around the DASH diet's core principles, featuring high-fiber, low-sodium recipes that support heart health, including a variety of breakfasts, meats, fish, snacks, soups, salads, and desserts.
The included meal plan promotes a diverse and balanced diet, emphasizing foods that lower blood pressure and boost heart health. While it doesn't include every recipe from the book, there's room for you to add sides, sauces, and beverages, tailoring meals to your tastes and health advice.

Use this plan as a flexible guide, combining recipes to suit your preferences. This approach keeps meals interesting and aligned with your health goals, proving that following the DASH diet can be flavorful and varied.
Start personalizing your meals for a heart-healthy eating experience.

Scan the QR Code below

to download your Shopping Lists in PDF format,

ready to make your meal planning even smoother

Week 1

Day	Breakfast	Lunch	Snack	Dinner	Dessert
1	Blueberry Protein Pancakes (3)	Baked Cod with Herbed Breadcrumbs (85)	Roasted Red Pepper Hummus with Carrot Sticks (26)	Grilled Lemon Herb Chicken (61)	Baked Pear with Cinnamon and Almonds (111)
2	Banana Nut Overnight Oats (2)	Beef and Broccoli Stir-Fry (63)	Pear Slices with Cottage Cheese (27)	Roasted Butternut Squash Salad (51)	Banana and Walnut Muffins (112)
3	Greek Yogurt with Kiwi Slices (20)	Lentil and Vegetable Soup (54)	Baked Kale Chips (28)	Lemon Dill Turkey Breast (71)	Chocolate Avocado Mousse (113)
4	Tomato and Basil Omelet (10)	Tomato Cucumber Salad with Dill (58)	Mixed Nuts (Unsalted) and Sliced Apple (32)	Salmon and Asparagus Foil Packets (86)	Apple Cinnamon Baked Oatmeal (114)
5	Breakfast Tofu Scramble (9)	Teriyaki Chicken (70)	Rice Cakes with Peanut Butter and Banana (30)	Gazpacho with Cucumber Salsa (59)	Berry and Yogurt Parfait (115)
6	Quinoa and Berry Breakfast Bowl (12)	Kale and Cranberry Salad (57)	Cucumber Slices with Greek Yogurt Dip (33)	Lemon Garlic Tilapia (88)	Baked Peaches with Almond Crumble (116)
7	Whole Wheat Crepes with Strawberries (16)	Roasted Garlic and White Bean Soup (60)	Greek Yogurt with Pomegranate Seeds (31)	Teriyaki Turkey Burgers (79)	Strawberry and Banana Popsicles (117)

Week 2

Day	Breakfast	Lunch	Snack	Dinner	Dessert
1	Overnight Chia Pudding with Mango (18)	Baked Trout with Almond Crust (96)	Sliced Bell Peppers with Guacamole (37)	Beef and Vegetable Stir-Fry (67)	Lemon Poppy Seed Muffins (118)
2	Almond and Date Breakfast Bars (24)	Chicken and Vegetable Stir-Fry Soup (52)	Air-Popped Popcorn (34)	Lemon Dill Mackerel (94)	Chocolate Covered Almonds (119)
3	Spinach and Mushroom Breakfast Quesadilla (1)	Herb-Crusted Pork Tenderloin (73)	Watermelon Cubes (38)	Caprese Salad with Balsamic Glaze (55)	Greek Yogurt and Berry Bark (120)
4	Whole Wheat French Toast with Berries (8)	Avocado and Quinoa Salad (56)	Pineapple and Cottage Cheese (39)	Teriyaki Chicken (70)	Coconut and Chia Seed Pudding (121)
5	Spinach and Tomato Breakfast Wrap (14)	Chicken and Mushroom Skillet (78)	Roasted Chickpeas (36)	Kale and Cranberry Salad (57)	Baked Apple Chips (122)
6	Peanut Butter and Banana Smoothie (5)	Beef and Pepper Stir-Fry (72)	Celery Sticks with Hummus and Raisins (43)	Tomato Cucumber Salad with Dill (58)	Mixed Fruit Sorbet (124)
7	Sweet Potato and Black Bean Hash (7)	Quinoa and Black Bean Salad (46)	Greek Yogurt with Papaya (41)	Balsamic Glazed Chicken Breast (76)	Pumpkin and Walnut Bites (125)

Week 3

Day	Breakfast	Lunch	Snack	Dinner	Dessert
1	Broccoli and Cheddar Frittata (13)	Roasted Beet and Goat Cheese Salad (47)	Sliced Mango with Lime (42)	Pork Chops with Apple and Cabbage (69)	Greek Yogurt and Berry Bark (120)
2	Quinoa and Spinach Breakfast Casserole (25)	Spinach and Chickpea Salad with Lemon Vinaigrette (48)	Almond Butter and Banana Slices (40)	Lean Beef and Vegetable Stir-Fry (75)	Coconut and Chia Seed Pudding (121)
3	Breakfast Muffin with Spinach and Feta (17)	Pork Stir-Fry with Broccoli and Snap Peas (77)	Cherry Tomato and Mozzarella Skewers (29)	Chicken and Vegetable Stir-Fry Soup (52)	Lemon Poppy Seed Muffins (118)
4	Oat Bran Cereal with Almond Milk (23)	Grilled Sardines with Herbs (92)	Greek Yogurt with Pomegranate Seeds (31)	Gazpacho with Cucumber Salsa (59)	Baked Pear with Cinnamon and Almonds (111)
5	Spinach and Feta Breakfast Pie (21)	Chicken and Mushroom Skillet (78)	Baked Kale Chips (28)	Turkey and Zucchini Meatballs (74)	Chocolate Avocado Mousse (113)
6	Breakfast Tacos with Black Beans and Avocado (22)	Seared Tuna with Sesame Seeds (97)	Rice Cakes with Peanut Butter and Banana (30)	Quinoa and Black Bean Salad (46)	Berry and Yogurt Parfait (115)
7	Cinnamon Raisin Oatmeal (15)	Lentil and Vegetable Soup (54)	Mixed Nuts (Unsalted) and Sliced Apple (32)	Swordfish and Vegetable Kebabs (95)	Banana and Walnut Muffins (112)

Week 4

Day	Breakfast	Lunch	Snack	Dinner	Dessert
1	Tomato and Basil Omelet (10)	Roasted Garlic and White Bean Soup (60)	Sliced Bell Peppers with Guacamole (37)	Teriyaki Turkey Burgers (79)	Banana and Walnut Muffins (112)
2	Almond Butter and Apple Sandwich (11)	Lemon Dill Turkey Breast (71)	Pineapple and Cottage Cheese (39)	Caprese Salad with Balsamic Glaze (55)	Chocolate Covered Almonds (119)
3	Quinoa and Berry Breakfast Bowl (12)	Spinach and Pomegranate Salad (53)	Watermelon Cubes (38)	Beef and Pepper Stir-Fry (72)	Greek Yogurt and Berry Bark (120)
4	Broccoli and Cheddar Frittata (13)	Teriyaki Chicken (70)	Celery Sticks with Hummus and Raisins (43)	Baked Trout with Almond Crust (96)	Pumpkin and Walnut Bites (125)
5	Spinach and Mushroom Breakfast Quesadilla (1)	Tomato Cucumber Salad with Dill (58)	Roasted Chickpeas (36)	Chicken and Mushroom Skillet (78)	Mixed Fruit Sorbet (124)
6	Peanut Butter and Banana Smoothie (5)	Lemon Buttered Catfish (98)	Greek Yogurt with Papaya (41)	Avocado and Quinoa Salad (56)	Coconut and Chia Seed Pudding (121)
7	Sweet Potato and Black Bean Hash (7)	Turkey and Zucchini Meatballs (74)	Greek Yogurt with Pomegranate Seeds (31)	Tuna and Cucumber Roll-Ups (93)	Lemon Poppy Seed Muffins (118)

Week 5

Day	Breakfast	Lunch	Snack	Dinner	Dessert
1	Banana Nut Overnight Oats (2)	Chicken and Vegetable Stir-Fry Soup (52)	Cherry Tomato and Mozzarella Skewers (29)	Grilled Lemon Herb Chicken (61)	Berry and Yogurt Parfait (115)
2	Spinach and Tomato Breakfast Wrap (14)	Greek Quinoa Salad (50)	Sliced Mango with Lime (42)	Baked Cod with Herbed Breadcrumbs (85)	Chocolate Avocado Mousse (113)
3	Whole Wheat French Toast with Berries (8)	Teriyaki Turkey Burgers (79)	Rice Cakes with Peanut Butter and Banana (30)	Lemon Garlic Chicken Thighs (68)	Baked Pear with Cinnamon and Almonds (111)
4	Breakfast Tacos with Black Beans and Avocado (22)	Baked Mahi-Mahi with Lemon Butter (83)	Mixed Nuts (Unsalted) and Sliced Apple (32)	Mushroom Barley Soup (49)	Greek Yogurt and Berry Bark (120)
5	Quinoa and Spinach Breakfast Casserole (25)	Gazpacho with Cucumber Salsa (59)	Watermelon Cubes (38)	Beef and Vegetable Stir-Fry (67)	Pumpkin and Walnut Bites (125)
6	Peanut Butter and Banana Smoothie (5)	Herb-Crusted Pork Tenderloin (73)	Cucumber Slices with Greek Yogurt Dip (33)	Caprese Salad with Balsamic Glaze (55)	Strawberry and Banana Popsicles (117)
7	Sweet Potato and Black Bean Hash (7)	Lentil and Vegetable Soup (54)	Roasted Chickpeas (36)	Pork Stir-Fry with Broccoli and Snap Peas (77)	Lemon Poppy Seed Muffins (118)

Week 6

Day	Breakfast	Lunch	Snack	Dinner	Dessert
1	Blueberry Protein Pancakes (3)	Turkey and Zucchini Meatballs (74)	Sliced Bell Peppers with Guacamole (37)	Lemon Dill Turkey Breast (71)	Banana and Walnut Muffins (112)
2	Almond and Date Breakfast Bars (24)	Chicken and Vegetable Stir-Fry Soup (52)	Air-Popped Popcorn (34)	Seared Scallops with Spinach and Tomato (89)	Mixed Fruit Sorbet (124)
3	Greek Yogurt with Kiwi Slices (20)	Spinach and Chickpea Salad with Lemon Vinaigrette (48)	Pineapple and Cottage Cheese (39)	Beef and Pepper Stir-Fry (72)	Coconut and Chia Seed Pudding (121)
4	Spinach and Mushroom Breakfast Quesadilla (1)	Teriyaki Chicken (70)	Mixed Nuts (Unsalted) and Sliced Apple (32)	Roasted Butternut Squash Salad (51)	Baked Peaches with Almond Crumble (116)
5	Breakfast Muffin with Spinach and Feta (17)	Avocado and Quinoa Salad (56)	Cherry Tomato and Mozzarella Skewers (29)	Lemon Garlic Tilapia (88)	Chocolate Covered Almonds (119)
6	Banana Nut Overnight Oats (2)	Teriyaki Turkey Burgers (79)	Rice Cakes with Peanut Butter and Banana (30)	Chicken and Mushroom Skillet (78)	Greek Yogurt and Berry Bark (120)
7	Quinoa and Berry Breakfast Bowl (12)	Baked Cod with Herbed Breadcrumbs (85)	Greek Yogurt with Papaya (41)	Tomato Cucumber Salad with Dill (58)	Strawberry and Banana Popsicles (117)

Week 7

Day	Breakfast	Lunch	Snack	Dinner	Dessert
1	Broccoli and Cheddar Frittata (13)	Salmon and Asparagus Foil Packets (86)	Watermelon Cubes (38)	Pork Chops with Apple and Cabbage (69)	Greek Yogurt and Berry Bark (120)
2	Quinoa and Spinach Breakfast Casserole (25)	Chicken and Mushroom Skillet (78)	Almond Butter and Banana Slices (40)	Gazpacho with Cucumber Salsa (59)	Coconut and Chia Seed Pudding (121)
3	Oat Bran Cereal with Almond Milk (23)	Lentil and Vegetable Soup (54)	Mixed Nuts (Unsalted) and Sliced Apple (32)	Lemon Buttered Catfish (98)	Baked Pear with Cinnamon and Almonds (111)
4	Almond and Date Breakfast Bars (24)	Caprese Salad with Balsamic Glaze (55)	Baked Kale Chips (28)	Teriyaki Turkey Burgers (79)	Chocolate Avocado Mousse (113)
5	Peanut Butter and Banana Smoothie (5)	Greek Quinoa Salad (50)	Sliced Bell Peppers with Guacamole (37)	Tuna and White Bean Salad with Lemon Dressing (87)	Berry and Yogurt Parfait (115)
6	Blueberry Protein Pancakes (3)	Lean Beef and Vegetable Stir-Fry (75)	Rice Cakes with Peanut Butter and Banana (30)	Spinach and Pomegranate Salad (53)	Pumpkin and Walnut Bites (125)
7	Spinach and Tomato Breakfast Wrap (14)	Chicken and Vegetable Stir-Fry Soup (52)	Cucumber Slices with Greek Yogurt Dip (33)	Balsamic Glazed Chicken Breast (76)	Strawberry and Banana Popsicles (117)

Week 8

Day	Breakfast	Lunch	Snack	Dinner	Dessert
1	Whole Wheat French Toast with Berries (8)	Teriyaki Turkey Burgers (79)	Sliced Bell Peppers with Guacamole (37)	Roasted Garlic and White Bean Soup (60)	Banana and Walnut Muffins (112)
2	Banana Nut Overnight Oats (2)	Caprese Salad with Balsamic Glaze (55)	Pineapple and Cottage Cheese (39)	Lemon Dill Turkey Breast (71)	Chocolate Covered Almonds (119)
3	Quinoa and Berry Breakfast Bowl (12)	Beef and Pepper Stir-Fry (72)	Watermelon Cubes (38)	Spinach and Pomegranate Salad (53)	Greek Yogurt and Berry Bark (120)
4	Sweet Potato and Black Bean Hash (7)	Avocado and Quinoa Salad (56)	Celery Sticks with Hummus and Raisins (43)	Swordfish and Vegetable Kebabs (95)	Baked Pear with Cinnamon and Almonds (111)
5	Spinach and Mushroom Breakfast Quesadilla (1)	Chicken and Mushroom Skillet (78)	Roasted Chickpeas (36)	Tomato Cucumber Salad with Dill (58)	Mixed Fruit Sorbet (124)
6	Peanut Butter and Banana Smoothie (5)	Tuna and Cucumber Roll-Ups (93)	Greek Yogurt with Papaya (41)	Teriyaki Chicken (70)	Coconut and Chia Seed Pudding (121)
7	Banana Nut Overnight Oats (2)	Quinoa and Black Bean Salad (46)	Greek Yogurt with Pomegranate Seeds (31)	Baked Trout with Almond Crust (96)	Lemon Poppy Seed Muffins (118)

Week 9

Day	Breakfast	Lunch	Snack	Dinner	Dessert
1	Spinach and Mushroom Breakfast Quesadilla (1)	Greek Quinoa Salad (50)	Mixed Berries with Greek Yogurt (44)	Grilled Lemon Herb Chicken (61)	Chocolate Avocado Mousse (113)
2	Blueberry Protein Pancakes (3)	Lentil and Vegetable Soup (54)	Pear Slices with Cottage Cheese (27)	Baked Cod with Herbed Breadcrumbs (85)	Berry and Yogurt Parfait (115)
3	Quinoa and Berry Breakfast Bowl (12)	Baked Snapper with Citrus Glaze (90)	Roasted Chickpeas (36)	Teriyaki Chicken (70)	Baked Peaches with Almond Crumble (116)
4	Overnight Chia Pudding with Mango (18)	Roasted Beet and Goat Cheese Salad (47)	Cherry Tomato and Mozzarella Skewers (29)	Beef and Vegetable Stir-Fry (67)	Lemon Poppy Seed Muffins (118)
5	Almond Butter and Apple Sandwich (11)	Beef and Pepper Stir-Fry (72)	Rice Cakes with Peanut Butter and Banana (30)	Lemon Dill Turkey Breast (71)	Greek Yogurt and Berry Bark (120)
6	Banana Nut Overnight Oats (2)	Chicken and Vegetable Stir-Fry Soup (52)	Cucumber Slices with Greek Yogurt Dip (33)	Tomato Cucumber Salad with Dill (58)	Strawberry and Banana Popsicles (117)
7	Breakfast Tacos with Black Beans and Avocado (22)	Teriyaki Turkey Burgers (79)	Mixed Nuts (Unsalted) and Sliced Apple (32)	Balsamic Glazed Chicken Breast (76)	Mixed Fruit Sorbet (124)

Week 10

Day	Breakfast	Lunch	Snack	Dinner	Dessert
1	Spinach and Tomato Breakfast Wrap (14)	Swordfish and Vegetable Kebabs (95)	Watermelon Cubes (38)	Lean Beef and Vegetable Stir-Fry (75)	Chocolate Covered Almonds (119)
2	Whole Wheat Crepes with Strawberries (16)	Chicken and Vegetable Stir-Fry Soup (52)	Greek Yogurt with Pomegranate Seeds (31)	Seared Tuna with Sesame Seeds (97)	Banana and Walnut Muffins (112)
3	Sweet Potato and Black Bean Hash (7)	Beef and Asparagus Stir-Fry (80)	Pineapple and Cottage Cheese (39)	Kale and Cranberry Salad (57)	Coconut and Chia Seed Pudding (121)
4	Quinoa and Spinach Breakfast Casserole (25)	Spinach and Chickpea Salad with Lemon Vinaigrette (48)	Mixed Nuts (Unsalted) and Sliced Apple (32)	Beef and Pepper Stir-Fry (72)	Pumpkin and Walnut Bites (125)
5	Breakfast Muffin with Spinach and Feta (17)	Teriyaki Turkey Burgers (79)	Cherry Tomato and Mozzarella Skewers (29)	Lemon Garlic Tilapia (88)	Greek Yogurt and Berry Bark (120)
6	Peanut Butter and Banana Smoothie (5)	Gazpacho with Cucumber Salsa (59)	Baked Kale Chips (28)	Chicken and Mushroom Skillet (78)	Strawberry and Banana Popsicles (117)
7	Greek Yogurt with Kiwi Slices (20)	Teriyaki Chicken (70)	Greek Yogurt with Papaya (41)	Avocado and Quinoa Salad (56)	Cranberry and Orange Smoothie (127)

Week 11

Day	Breakfast	Lunch	Snack	Dinner	Dessert
1	Banana Nut Overnight Oats (2)	Caprese Salad with Balsamic Glaze (55)	Roasted Red Pepper Hummus with Carrot Sticks (26)	Teriyaki Chicken (70)	Baked Pear with Cinnamon and Almonds (111)
2	Blueberry Protein Pancakes (3)	Turkey and Spinach Stuffed Mushrooms (62)	Pear Slices with Cottage Cheese (27)	Baked Cod with Herbed Breadcrumbs (85)	Chocolate Avocado Mousse (113)
3	Veggie Breakfast Burrito (6)	Lemon Buttered Catfish (98)	Baked Kale Chips (28)	Beef and Pepper Stir-Fry (72)	Apple Cinnamon Baked Oatmeal (114)
4	Almond Butter and Apple Sandwich (11)	Chicken and Veggie Skewers with Tzatziki (65)	Greek Yogurt with Pomegranate Seeds (31)	Avocado and Quinoa Salad (56)	Berry and Yogurt Parfait (115)
5	Spinach and Tomato Breakfast Wrap (14)	Roasted Garlic and White Bean Soup (60)	Mixed Nuts and Sliced Apple (32)	Teriyaki Turkey Burgers (79)	Baked Peaches with Almond Crumble (116)
6	Breakfast Tacos with Black Beans and Avocado (22)	Beef and Vegetable Stir-Fry (67)	Cucumber Slices with Greek Yogurt Dip (33)	Chicken and Vegetable Stir-Fry Soup (52)	Lemon Poppy Seed Muffins (118)
7	Oat Bran Cereal with Almond Milk (23)	Lemon Garlic Chicken Thighs (68)	Watermelon Cubes (38)	Lemon Buttered Catfish (98)	Coconut and Chia Seed Pudding (121)

Week 12

Day	Breakfast	Lunch	Snack	Dinner	Dessert
1	Whole Wheat French Toast with Berries (8)	Quinoa and Black Bean Salad (46)	Pear Slices with Cottage Cheese (27)	Seared Scallops with Spinach and Tomato (89)	Chocolate Avocado Mousse (113)
2	Banana Nut Overnight Oats (2)	Pork Tenderloin with Mustard Sauce (64)	Baked Kale Chips (28)	Lemon Dill Turkey Breast (71)	Berry and Yogurt Parfait (115)
3	Quinoa and Berry Breakfast Bowl (12)	Mushroom Barley Soup (49)	Greek Yogurt with Pomegranate Seeds (31)	Pork Chops with Apple and Cabbage (69)	Strawberry and Banana Popsicles (117)
4	Breakfast Tofu Scramble (9)	Teriyaki Chicken (70)	Mixed Nuts and Sliced Apple (32)	Tuna and Cucumber Roll-Ups (93)	Coconut and Chia Seed Pudding (121)
5	Almond Butter and Apple Sandwich (11)	Spinach and Pomegranate Salad (53)	Roasted Chickpeas (36)	Seared Tuna with Sesame Seeds (97)	Baked Apple Chips (122)
6	Spinach and Tomato Breakfast Wrap (14)	Salmon and Asparagus Foil Packets (86)	Watermelon Cubes (38)	Beef and Vegetable Stir-Fry (67)	Mixed Fruit Sorbet (124)
7	Cinnamon Raisin Oatmeal (15)	Teriyaki Turkey Burgers (79)	Greek Yogurt with Papaya (41)	Roasted Beet and Goat Cheese Salad (47)	Pumpkin and Walnut Bites (125)

Conversion Table

Volume Equivalents (Liquid)

US Standard	US Standard (ounces)	Metric (approximate)
2 tablespoons	1 fl. oz.	30 mL
¼ cup	2 fl. oz.	60 mL
½ cup	4 fl. oz.	120 mL
1 cup	8 fl. oz.	240 mL
1½ cups	12 fl. oz.	355 mL
2 cups or 1 pint	16 fl. oz.	475 mL
4 cups or 1 quart	32 fl. oz.	1 L
1 gallon	128 fl. oz.	4 L

Volume Equivalents (Dry)

US Standard	Metric (approximate)
⅛ teaspoon	0.5 mL
¼ teaspoon	1 mL
½ teaspoon	2 mL
¾ teaspoon	4 mL
1 teaspoon	5 mL
1 tablespoon	15 mL
¼ cup	59 mL
⅓ cup	79 mL
½ cup	118 mL
⅔ cup	156 mL
¾ cup	177 mL
1 cup	235 mL
2 cups or 1 pint	475 mL
3 cups	700 mL
4 cups or 1 quart	1 L

Oven Temperatures

Fahrenheit (F)	Celsius (C) (approximate)
250°F	120°C
300°F	150°C
325°F	165°C
350°F	180°C
375°F	190°C
400°F	200°C
425°F	220°C
450°F	230°C

Weight Equivalents

US Standard	Metric (approximate)
1 tablespoon	15 g
½ ounce	15 g
1 ounce	30 g
2 ounces	60 g
4 ounces	115 g
8 ounces	225 g
12 ounces	340 g
16 ounces or 1 pound	455 g

Index

Air-Popped Popcorn; 34
Almond and Date Breakfast Bars; 29
Almond Butter and Apple Sandwich; 21
Almond Butter and Banana Slices; 36
Apple Cinnamon Baked Oatmeal; 84
Apple Cinnamon Rice Cakes; 38
Avocado and Quinoa Salad; 45
Baked Apple Chips; 89
Baked Cod with Herbed Breadcrumbs; 66
Baked Haddock with Lemon Pepper; 75
Baked Kale Chips; 32
Baked Mahi-Mahi with Lemon Butter; 65
Baked Peaches with Almond Crumble; 86
Baked Pear with Cinnamon and Almonds; 83
Baked Snapper with Citrus Glaze; 69
Baked Trout with Almond Crust; 73
Baked Turkey Meatloaf; 52
Balsamic Glazed Chicken Breast; 59
Banana and Walnut Muffins; 83
Banana Nut Overnight Oats; 16
Beef and Asparagus Stir-Fry; 62
Beef and Broccoli Stir-Fry; 50
Beef and Pepper Stir-Fry; 56
Beef and Vegetable Stir-Fry; 53
Berry and Yogurt Parfait; 85
Blueberry Protein Pancakes; 17
Breakfast Muffin with Spinach and Feta; 25
Breakfast Tacos with Black Beans and Avocado; 27
Breakfast Tofu Scramble; 20
Broccoli and Cheddar Frittata; 22
Brown Rice and Black Beans; 78
Canned Mackerel Salad; 70
Caprese Salad with Balsamic Glaze; 45
Celery Sticks with Hummus and Raisins; 37
Cherry and Pomegranate Iced Tea; 93
Cherry Tomato and Mozzarella Skewers; 32
Chicken and Mushroom Skillet; 61
Chicken and Vegetable Stir-Fry Soup; 43
Chicken and Veggie Skewers with Tzatziki; 51
Chocolate Avocado Mousse; 84
Chocolate Covered Almonds; 87
Cilantro Lime Brown Rice; 81
Cinnamon Raisin Oatmeal; 23
Coconut and Chia Seed Pudding; 88
Cottage Cheese and Pineapple Bowl; 26

Cranberry and Orange Smoothie; 92
Cucumber and Mint Cooler; 93
Cucumber Slices with Greek Yogurt Dip; 34
Edamame; 34
Gazpacho with Cucumber Salsa; 47
Greek Quinoa Salad; 42
Greek Yogurt and Berry Bark; 88
Greek Yogurt with Kiwi Slices; 26
Greek Yogurt with Papaya; 37
Greek Yogurt with Pomegranate Seeds; 33
Grilled Halibut with Mango Salsa; 64
Grilled Lemon Herb Chicken; 49
Grilled Sardines with Herbs; 70
Herbal Infusion with Mint and Ginger; 92
Herb-Crusted Pork Tenderloin; 57
Kale and Cranberry Salad; 46
Kiwi and Spinach Smoothie; 94
Lean Beef and Vegetable Stir-Fry; 59
Lemon Buttered Catfish; 74
Lemon Dill Mackerel; 72
Lemon Dill Turkey Breast; 56
Lemon Garlic Chicken Thighs; 54
Lemon Garlic Tilapia; 68
Lemon Poppy Seed Muffins; 87
Lentil and Vegetable Soup; 44
Mashed Butternut Squash; 80
Mixed Berries with Greek Yogurt; 38
Mixed Fruit Sorbet; 90
Mixed Nuts (Unsalted) and Sliced Apple; 33
Mushroom Barley Soup; 41
Oat Bran Cereal with Almond Milk; 28
Overnight Chia Pudding with Mango; 25
Peanut Butter and Banana Smoothie; 18
Pear Slices with Cottage Cheese; 31
Pineapple and Coconut Frozen Yogurt; 89
Pineapple and Cottage Cheese; 36
Poached Eggs with Salsa; 17
Pork Chops with Apple and Cabbage; 54
Pork Stir-Fry with Broccoli and Snap Peas; 60
Pork Tenderloin with Mustard Sauce; 51
Pumpkin and Walnut Bites; 90
Quinoa and Berry Breakfast Bowl; 22
Quinoa and Black Bean Salad; 39
Quinoa and Spinach Breakfast Casserole; 29
Quinoa and Vegetable Pilaf; 77

Rice Cakes with Peanut Butter and Banana; 33
Roasted Beet and Goat Cheese Salad; 40
Roasted Brussels Sprouts with Balsamic Glaze; 82
Roasted Butternut Squash Salad; 42
Roasted Cauliflower with Turmeric; 77
Roasted Chickpeas; 35
Roasted Eggplant with Tahini Sauce; 79
Roasted Garlic and White Bean Soup; 48
Roasted Red Pepper Hummus with Carrot Sticks; 31
Salmon and Asparagus Foil Packets; 67
Sardine and Olive Tapenade; 75
Sautéed Spinach with Pine Nuts; 80
Sautéed Swiss Chard with Garlic; 78
Seared Scallops with Spinach and Tomato; 68
Seared Tuna with Sesame Seeds; 73
Shrimp and Spinach Salad; 65
Sliced Bell Peppers with Guacamole; 35
Sliced Mango with Lime; 37
Spinach and Chickpea Salad with Lemon Vinaigrette; 40
Spinach and Feta Breakfast Pie; 27
Spinach and Mushroom Breakfast Quesadilla; 16
Spinach and Pomegranate Salad; 44
Spinach and Tomato Breakfast Wrap; 23
Steamed Artichokes with Lemon Butter; 81
Strawberry and Banana Popsicles; 86
Sweet Potato and Black Bean Hash; 19
Swordfish and Vegetable Kebabs; 72
Teriyaki Chicken; 55
Teriyaki Turkey Burgers; 62
Tomato and Basil Omelet; 21
Tomato Cucumber Salad with Dill; 47
Tuna and Cucumber Roll-Ups; 71
Tuna and White Bean Salad with Lemon Dressing; 67
Tuna Salad Lettuce Wraps; 64
Turkey and Spinach Stuffed Mushrooms; 49
Turkey and Zucchini Meatballs; 58
Veggie Breakfast Burrito; 18
Watermelon Cubes; 36
Whole Wheat Crepes with Strawberries; 24
Whole Wheat French Toast with Berries; 20

BONUSES

"Every Step Counts"

Elevate your path to better health!

Scan this QR Code to access your exclusive bonus, 'Every Step Counts' and discover the ideal physical activities to complement your DASH Diet journey.

Embrace wellness with every step on this journey!

"Empowering Mindset - Pathways to Holistic Health and Resilience"

Transform your approach to health with positive thinking.

Scan the QR Code to download 'Empowering Mindset - Pathways to Holistic Health and Resilience' a pivotal guide to strengthening your mindset as you embark on the DASH Diet journey.

Discover the power of resilience and holistic wellness.

Conclusions and Recommendations

Maintaining a healthy lifestyle is a multifaceted journey that involves making informed choices about your diet, incorporating regular physical activity, and nurturing a positive mindset. In this concluding section, we will underscore the significance of these three essential elements and provide suggestions for achieving a balanced and sustainable approach to overall well-being.

The Importance of the Meal Plan

A well-structured meal plan is the cornerstone of a healthy lifestyle. It provides a framework for making nutritious food choices, controlling portion sizes, and managing calorie intake. Here are some essential insights highlighting the significance of a meal plan:

1. **Nutrient Balance**: a thoughtfully designed meal plan ensures that you receive a balanced intake of essential nutrients like vitamins, minerals, protein, carbohydrates, and healthy fats. This equilibrium aids in numerous body functions, ranging from producing energy to maintaining immune system health.
2. **Blood Sugar Management**: planning meals that incorporate complex carbohydrates, lean proteins, and fiber-rich foods helps stabilize blood sugar levels. This is crucial for preventing energy spikes and crashes and reducing the risk of type 2 diabetes.
3. **Weight Management**: a well-structured meal plan supports weight management goals. By managing portion sizes and opting for nutrient-dense foods, you can attain and sustain a healthy weight, thereby diminishing the risk of health issues associated with obesity.
4. **Consistency**: having a meal plan in place promotes dietary consistency. Consistency is essential for creating long-term habits that contribute to overall health and well-being.
5. **Healthy Food Choices**: a meal plan encourages you to make healthier food choices. It helps you avoid impulsive and less nutritious options, particularly when dining out or during busy days.

Recommendations for Meal Planning

- Collaborate with a registered dietitian or nutritionist to develop a customized meal plan that aligns with your dietary preferences, lifestyle, and health goals.
- Focus on whole, minimally processed foods. Incorporate plenty of fruits, whole grains, vegetables, lean proteins, and healthy fats into your meals.
- Plan your meals and snacks in advance to reduce the likelihood of making unhealthy food choices when you're hungry and pressed for time.
- Experiment with new recipes and flavors to keep your meal plan interesting and enjoyable.
- Be flexible and open to adjustments as your dietary needs and preferences evolve over time.

The Importance of Combining the Diet with Physical Exercises

A healthy diet is essential, but it's only part of the equation for overall well-being. Physical activity plays a vital role in maintaining good health and preventing chronic diseases. Here's why combining a balanced diet with regular exercise is crucial:

1. **Weight Management**: exercise helps burn calories, contributing to weight management and supporting a healthy body composition. It complements dietary efforts by increasing the energy expenditure side of the equation.
2. **Cardiovascular Health**: physical activity strengthens the heart and improves circulation. Regular physical activity can contribute to lowering blood pressure, decreasing the risk of heart disease, and enhancing overall cardiovascular fitness.
3. **Muscle and Bone Health**: regular exercise supports muscle development and helps maintain bone density, reducing the risk of osteoporosis and frailty as you age.
4. **Mental Health**: exercise has profound effects on mental well-being. It reduces stress, anxiety, and depression while promoting positive mood and better cognitive function.
5. **Energy and Stamina**: engaging in physical activity increases energy levels and stamina, enhancing your ability to perform daily tasks and activities.
6. **Longevity**: numerous studies have shown that regular exercise is associated with increased life expectancy and a higher quality of life in later years.

Recommendations for Combining Diet with Physical Exercise

- Discover physical activities that you like to integrate exercise into your routine sustainably. It could be anything from walking and cycling to dancing or team sports.
- Strive for a minimum of 150 minutes of moderate-intensity aerobic exercise or 75 minutes of vigorous-intensity aerobic exercise each week, in accordance with health recommendations.
- Include strength training workouts at least twice a week to develop and preserve muscle mass.
- Create a balanced fitness plan that includes cardiovascular, strength, flexibility, and balance exercises to address all aspects of physical health.
- Before initiating a new exercise program, especially if you have preexisting health conditions or concerns, consult with a healthcare provider or fitness professional.

The Importance of Not Getting Discouraged and Always Maintaining a Positive Mindset

Maintaining a positive mindset is a fundamental aspect of a healthy lifestyle. Maintaining motivation and commitment to your health goals can be challenging, but cultivating a positive outlook can make a significant difference. Here's why it's essential and some recommendations:

1. **Resilience**: a positive mindset enhances resilience, enabling you to rebound from setbacks and stay on course, even in the face of challenges.
2. **Motivation**: positivity fuels motivation. When you approach your health goals with optimism and a belief in your ability to succeed, you're more likely to stay committed and take consistent action.
3. **Stress Reduction**: maintaining a positive mindset reduces stress and its negative effects on your body. Lower stress levels promote better overall health and well-being.
4. **Self-compassion**: positivity includes self-compassion and self-acceptance. It's essential to treat yourself with kindness and forgiveness, especially when you face setbacks or make mistakes.
5. **Improved Relationships**: a positive attitude can improve your relationships with others, fostering a supportive environment that encourages healthy habits.

Recommendations for Maintaining a Positive Mindset

- Incorporate mindfulness and meditation into your routine to alleviate stress and enhance emotional resilience.
- Establish realistic and achievable goals for your health journey, celebrating small victories along the way.
- Envelop yourself in a supportive network of friends and family who not only encourage your efforts but also share similar health goals.
- Use positive affirmations and self-talk to boost self-esteem and reinforce your commitment to a healthy lifestyle.
- Seek professional help or counseling if you struggle with persistent negative thoughts or mental health issues.

In conclusion, a healthy lifestyle is a holistic endeavor that involves a well-structured meal plan, regular physical exercise, and a positive mindset. These three elements work synergistically to promote overall well-being, prevent chronic diseases, and enhance the quality of life. By prioritizing these aspects and making them a consistent part of your daily routine, you can achieve and maintain optimal health for years to come. Remember that small, sustainable changes can lead to significant improvements in your health and overall quality of life.

Made in United States
Troutdale, OR
05/30/2024